WE NEED TO TALK

WE NEED TO TALK

DR TONY HOLOHAN

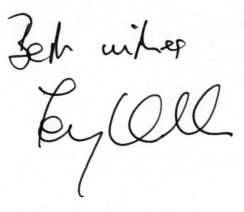

eriu

First published by Eriu
An imprint of Black & White Publishing Group
A Bonnier Books UK company

4th Floor, Victoria House,
Bloomsbury Square,
London, WC1B 4DA

Owned by Bonnier Books
Sveavägen 56, Stockholm, Sweden

– @eriu_books
– @eriubooks

Hardback – 978-1-80418-249-9
Ebook – 978-1-80418-380-9

'Clearances' from *The Haw Lantern* by Seamus Heaney has been reproduced
with the permission of Faber and Faber Ltd.

A CIP catalogue of this book is available from the British Library.

Typeset by IDSUK (Data Connection) Ltd
Printed and bound by Clays Ltd, Elcograf S.p.A

1 3 5 7 9 10 8 6 4 2

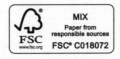

Every reasonable effort has been made to trace copyright holders of material
reproduced in this book, but if any have been inadvertently overlooked
the publishers would be glad to hear from them.

Eriu is an imprint of Bonnier Books UK
www.bonnierbooks.co.uk

For Emer, Clodagh and Ronan with love

Contents

Preface   ix

Prologue   x

Chapter One: Beginnings   1

Chapter Two: UCD and Emer   10

Chapter Three: UCD and After   18

Chapter Four: A Hard Lesson Learned   28

Chapter Five: Early Married Life   34

Chapter Six: Deputy Chief Medical Officer   43

Chapter Seven: Chief Medical Officer   53

Chapter Eight: Swine Flu   59

Chapter Nine: Emer's Diagnosis   66

Chapter Ten: Everything Changes   75

Chapter Eleven: Getting on with Life   89

Chapter Twelve: CervicalCheck: First Knowledge   98

Chapter Thirteen: CervicalCheck: Second Stage   114

Chapter Fourteen: The Abortion Referendum   124

Chapter Fifteen: Difficult Times   136

Chapter Sixteen: The Arrival of Covid   149

Chapter Seventeen: Covid: Our First Case 169

Chapter Eighteen: Covid: 'The Hammer and the Dance' 177

Chapter Nineteen: Covid: Day to Day 196

Chapter Twenty: Covid: The End in Sight 202

Chapter Twenty-One: Emer's Last Days 217

Chapter Twenty-Two: Emer's Funeral 222

Chapter Twenty-Three: Time To Go 234

Chapter Twenty-Four: My Secondment 245

Chapter Twenty-Five: Leaving 255

Chapter Twenty-Six: Difficult Conversations 267

Acknowledgments 276

Preface

With the opportunity I have to write this book, I want to tell Emer's story. So much of my career has been very public, but I was never on my own in any of it. Emer was with me through it all. Her story is part of my story, but her story is also her own story. She spoke to me about her wish to have her story told and she addressed this in the letters she left for me after her death. She hoped that her story might help others. That is what she wanted.

The book also tells my story. It is a story of one life with one journey. My personal and professional experiences were not separate from one another. My story is based on my recollections. It is not an exhaustive chronicle of every event and issue. Passions and feelings are less easily forgotten. I have done my best to recount them.

Prologue

Friday 10 January 2020
Dillinger's restaurant, Ranelagh

I remember the evening of 10 January 2020 very clearly. It was my daughter Clodagh's 19th birthday. Clodagh loves Christmas. So much so that I used to think she wouldn't get through Christmas ending and school returning, except for the fact that her birthday is on 10 January. This softens the blow for her.

We usually celebrated in the same way: a family dinner in a local restaurant. Dillinger's has often been our choice. It's close enough to where we live, and that became more important as Emer's illness progressed. That year, she was quite a bit more unwell even than she had been.

By then, we were into what in my mind I have characterised as the 'second four years' of Emer's illness. She had been diagnosed with multiple myeloma in 2012. Myeloma is incurable. Once that diagnosis is given, it is only a matter of time. And often, not very much time. Three or four years would be an average survival time, certainly at the stage at which Emer had been diagnosed.

Those 'second four years' were very different in quality to the previous four. At first, she had been relatively well, despite the disease and the treatment it required. Even with the debilitating effects of myeloma, she had been able to do things for herself, do things for and with the children, and continue with her work as a public health doctor.

During the second four years, she was in even more pain, and it was harder to manage. She had new lesions from the disease more often, and they caused greater side effects and localised problems. Gradually, she was losing her independence. She was no longer able to work or drive, and bit by bit she was losing the ability to care for herself.

But she had beaten the odds. She had fought so hard for every extra year.

There we were, that Friday night. Emer, Clodagh, Ronan and me. Still together, despite everything. That was something, I knew, that was very precious. Clodagh turned 19 that day. Emer hadn't believed she would live long enough to see her to 18, and yet here she was.

But instead of fully appreciating the wonder of this, I was preoccupied.

I had been picking up reports of a new coronavirus in a place called Wuhan in China. There wasn't very much information yet. A lot of the conversations I was having with public health colleagues were vague: 'What is this thing?'; 'What are you seeing?'

I had been Chief Medical Officer for twelve years by then, and in that time I had been through a variety of public health crises. There was SARS, also a coronavirus. There was the dioxin scandal, something that threw me out into the media on literally my very first day as CMO. And in 2009 there was swine flu, a global pandemic.

So I had some experience. I had a clear understanding of what needed to be done in the event of a global incident. My mind was on how ready we were as a country, and on what else we needed to put in place.

I was also conscious that we were in the middle of a general election campaign. The election date had been set for early February. The impact of that on any government department is very significant. Frankly, almost everything shuts down. Legally, ministers are still in place – their positions are never vacant; there must always be a minister – but in practice, all new policy work stops and all ministerial duties come to a halt until a new person is appointed. Only essential emergency work takes place.

It was an opportunity, therefore, for us to take stock of plans. To focus on what needed to be done beyond the immediate. For me, this was specifically a time to make sure that we were properly prepared for what was coming.

That was my focus as I sat in Dillinger's on that Friday night.

I knew Covid-19 was going to be a problem. There was nothing about any of the early reports that gave me any reassurance. I knew we would be dealing directly with cases of this disease within a few weeks.

No one at that stage, however, could have known that Covid would become the defining public health emergency of our time – but I knew enough to know there would be trouble, and to be running through all the things I needed to do, make sure of and put in place before that came to pass, even while I looked at a menu, ordered food, ate and talked.

As I look back now, if I had known what was coming – had known how the next two years would unfold for all of us and for my family – I would have tried to put work from my mind and focus on the precious time we still had together.

By the time the emergency phase of the Covid pandemic passed, Emer was no longer with us. Ronan had done his Leaving Certificate, without Emer, but guided by her advice almost to the end. Clodagh had spent most of her first year in college, attending online for the final term. Both had been completely isolated from their friends for months at a time. And I had worked many seven-day weeks, while Emer grew sicker.

I look back now at the people sitting at that table, and I want to tell myself, 'Pay attention to what's in front of you now. Make the most of it. Because it's fragile.'

CHAPTER ONE

Beginnings

I CAN'T RECALL THE specific moment I decided I'd like to study medicine. In my latter years in secondary school, when people asked what I wanted to do, I would say medicine. Maybe that was because I thought I could get the points to get in. I wasn't especially studious, but I felt I could do well enough.

My understanding of what choosing medicine would mean was limited, to say the least. There were no doctors or health-care professionals in my family. My insights, such as they were, were mostly about hospitals. In part that would have come from television. I remember picking up on the drama of the emergency department and the urgency of surgery. I wouldn't have had any real understanding of general practice. My experiences as a patient were limited to the occasional visit for stitches and a tetanus injection, that kind of thing. Certainly, that's not what I had in mind when I thought about medicine.

I didn't worry that I didn't know what was ahead; but I made the decision to put medicine in UCD at the top of my CAO application. It may not have been a very well-informed decision, but in spite of that it has proved a good one.

* * *

My father, Liam, was born in Coon, near Castlecomer, in 1939, the youngest of 11, with three sisters and seven brothers. He was a garda. His first posting as a young garda, following his training in the Phoenix Park, was in Bailieboro, County Cavan. After that he was sent to Hollyfort, near Gorey, County Wexford. Some months later he was transferred to Howth, County Dublin, where he met my mother in 1965. She was Brigid Ryan, some years his junior, from near Cappamore in County Limerick, the eldest girl in a family of three sisters and two older brothers. When she met my father she was working in the Custom House as a young civil servant – a position she had to relinquish when they married in 1966.

I was born in Holles Street, Dublin in 1967. We lived in Grange Park, Baldoyle, next to the old racecourse. I started school in St Peter and Paul's (now St Laurence's) Primary School and have many happy memories from that time.

Dad was transferred from Dublin to Limerick in the 1970s so my mother could be closer to her ageing parents in Cappamore. That meant that I did most of my growing up in Limerick, in the Castletroy area, the eldest of six, and the only boy. My twin sisters, Aileen and Therese, born in 1968, are slightly less than a year younger than me. Irish triplets! Next, in order, are Breda, Sinead and Aoife; Aoife was the only one of us born in Limerick. Looking back, I'm sure raising six children on a garda's salary meant money was often tight, but somehow my parents managed, and we never felt we were short of money. There was always care and attention and love.

I don't recall being conscious of it, but because I was the eldest, and a boy, I was probably given privileges that my sisters didn't have. Not that the girls would have been restricted, but opportunities came my way that maybe did not come theirs. Certainly, as far as my sisters are concerned, that isn't even a question! They would say I got plenty of freedom that they didn't get. And not just freedom. They have a joke that my mother's parents – who lived in her old homeplace about 10 miles outside Limerick, near Cappamore – once sent £10 in an envelope as their Christmas present to us. And of that £10, there was £5 for me and £5 to be split between the girls. I don't think that actually happened, but they are adamant that it did.

What is true is that I was very close to my grandmother Ellen (*née* O'Rourke), better known as Babe, and she probably did spoil me. My grandfather was Thomas Ryan (Luke). All the Ryans in that part of Ireland are known by nicknames to distinguish them, so his was Luke. They were dairy farmers, and during my pre-teen years I would go to the farm near Cappamore quite a bit. My parents would visit every week with my sisters, but I spent many weekends and all my school holidays there for two or three years. I remember getting my first racing bike, a confirmation present from my parents, and how I used to cycle in and out to the farm by myself, about 10 miles each way. That was a great thrill – the independence of it. I remember being out on the farm for the whole summer for those pre-teen years, and I loved that.

My grandparents lived in a big old house that had been divided – in that Irish way – once the eldest son got married. This son, my uncle Paddy, was the one running the farm by the time I began to spend my time there. During those years, my grandfather died, but much of the work had already been passed on to Paddy.

Even more than the farming, I was keen on helping Paddy with the agricultural show that took place every year. This was the Cappamore Show, and my uncle was secretary of the committee for sixty-three years until he died in 2021. His job was to organise and run the event, and I loved helping him with that. He had a specially commissioned caravan at the back behind the house, and that was the HQ, where all the logistics happened. I can still remember the many different categories of competition. There were competitions for show animals, for art, baking, sewing and show jumping. I got to understand which competitions were under-subscribed; one was 'an arrangement of wild fruit'. So every year I picked some crab apples, sloes and haws and arranged them in moss on a biscuit tin lid . . . and won a prize!

The show was at the end of August, so preparations for the show would go on through the whole summer. Mornings were for milking the cows, and then, during the course of the day, show administration would take over. Some of it was pure drudgery. For example, all the animals had to have a number hung on them – a piece of white card attached by two pieces of string. So I would be punching holes in cards evening after evening, while watching TV, until my hands were blistered. It was basic work, but I loved knowing how everything was put together, how the day was made to happen, how the prizes were awarded, and everything that happened behind the scenes. Because of that, I came to appreciate what it took to organise these kinds of things, how much effort was put in by the local community. I think that was important to understand, and I'm grateful that I learned it in such an organic way.

At the event itself, there would be a couple of thousand people. Competitors, spectators, hawkers selling all manner of things. I would get a few quid for my efforts, and I'd be able to spend it on buying their wares. There were roulette tables – something I'd never seen before – also lucky dips, shooting and ring-throwing games where the target was a piece of wood with a crisp pound note and a watch tied to its base. Some years, RTÉ would show up to do a report, and I remember the sense of 'there are TV cameras here', which, for a child, felt like a big deal. One year, the show featured on the evening news.

Despite all that, I didn't see myself as being part of that rural community in Cappamore. I was living in Castletroy and I was going to the Christian Brothers school in Sexton Street. I was very clear that I was a city kid. I liked living in the city, going to school there and having easy access to the amenities we had in that part of Limerick City.

For a few years, the farm, and my grandmother and uncle, were very much the focus of my spare time, and then I suddenly lost interest in it. I suppose, like any teenager, my life became all about hanging out with friends, and I began to think more and more about moving on from Limerick.

* * *

My parents took in summer students for a few years. I remember a Spanish girl, Begoña, from Bilbao, who was with us for one summer, and then her brother Fernando came for a couple of summers in a row. After that a French girl, Frédérique, was with us for two summers.

The great thing about that was I got to go to France the year after she first came, to stay with her family. They lived in Lyon and had a summer house in the countryside, halfway between Lyon and the city of Saint-Étienne, which was famous because Michel Platini played for the city's football club. That was 1982, the year France made it to the World Cup semi-final, and he was their star player.

That was a fantastic, idyllic month. The family had a big garden with a swimming pool, which I jumped into every morning before breakfast. They also had a moped, which I learned to ride. Eventually. At my first attempt, much to the amusement of Frédérique and her family, I crashed it into a hedge. I hadn't realised you were supposed to let go of the throttle to slow down . . .

Frédérique was maybe a year older than me. I was probably very taken with her, and I'm perfectly sure she didn't have the slightest bit of interest in me! She was the youngest of four. There was an older sister who had kids and would come over for lunch on Sundays, and two older brothers, one of whom was a junior hospital doctor in one of the hospitals in Lyon. I thought he was the coolest thing since sliced bread. I was 15 at that stage, and he was about ten years older. He had a very pretty girlfriend, and he would show up with her in a Citroën Deux Chevaux. I had my first alcoholic drink, out with Frederique and her parents one evening; a watered-down glass of red wine. I still remember that first experience of feeling ever so slightly tipsy!

Looking back, I think Frédérique's brother probably had some influence on my choice of medicine as well. After all, where do we get our ideas of what to be, except by piecing together scraps and images from the people and experiences around us?

These scraps and fragments can come from anywhere, and their origin can be surprising. Sometimes things stay with you that you don't expect.

* * *

Our first house in Limerick was very close to what is now the University of Limerick (UL). Back then, it was two colleges – the National Institute of Higher Education (NIHE) and the National College of Physical Education (NCPE). We arrived from Dublin in 1973, and I remember my parents telling me before we left Dublin that there was a park across the road from this new house. In fact, it was a field that soon after we moved to Limerick was prepared for building houses that then didn't get built. It was left in quite a state – covered in piles of stone and rubble that we used to call 'the rocks' – but it was an exciting place to play.

Some years after we moved to Limerick, my mother did a course in Montessori teaching, and set up and ran her own playschool. The garage was converted into what we called the 'toy room', with little tables and chairs and shelves full of bright toys.

When I was in primary school, some Traveller families moved their caravans onto 'the rocks', and my mother would let the children come to the playroom to play with the toys. She would often feed them. I remember she used to give them some of her wonderful apple sponge. I believe she had a sense that 'these kids need to be looked after.' And she never suggested that we shouldn't play with these families, which I think was unusual for the time and place. I remember us going over to 'the rocks', and being in their caravans. It wasn't something I thought very much about. Two of the children ended up in our school, Monaleen National School, and one was in my class. My father recalls me asking him if I would be allowed to pay for his school tour so he could come with the rest of the class.

This would have been second class. I can still remember being teased about knowing him, and about my mother bringing these kids to our house. I didn't really understand why; it was mysterious to me, although it clearly made an impression, because it stayed with me as a memory, along with a strong sense of admiration for my mother.

In 1979, my parents bought a plot of land and built a house, about a mile further down the road. My mother took her playschool experience and skills further, to work with Limerick social services as a playschool teacher in some of the most deprived areas of the city. During these years, we would listen to my mother's stories about some of the children she encountered, the families they came from and the challenges they faced. She would talk about children with headlice – now, any child can get headlice, but these would be serious infestations that spoke of neglect and poor hygiene. Through hearing everything she told us about the experiences of children that were just so completely different to the experiences my sisters and I had growing up, I began to gain an awareness of inequality, and a growing understanding of social perspective. I began to realise that not everyone had the good fortune that I had in my family and community. I was increasingly aware of the unfairness of other people's circumstances and how that influenced their access to opportunities I took for granted.

The Christian Brothers school I went to in Sexton Street, Limerick City furthered that. Limerick is a small enough city, so all of human life was there. We had classmates from deprived city backgrounds, from the countryside; farmers' sons, business owners' sons. It was a good school that had a very broad social mix. I had great friends there, as well as a great group of friends who lived near me and who attended other schools in the city. Chris Lynch was with me throughout our time in Sexton Street, where his father Eric was a legendary English and history teacher.

I lost contact with many of these friends for years. I left school, left home and left Limerick, all at the same time, and inevitably we lost touch. By the early 1990s my grandparents had died and my dad had retired from the Gardaí. My parents made the decision to move to Kilkenny City where they built a B&B and ran that successfully for 25 years. A new career for them in my dad's home county. Other than one sister, Breda, who lives there, I no longer have any direct link to Limerick.

Strangely, in more recent years and especially during Covid, I found myself back in contact with some of my old friends from Limerick. I think we all became more reflective for a time – examining our friendships, our family, our past, which relationships we valued. I certainly did, and as part of that process, some of these old school friends have come back into my life, which has been a wonderful and unexpected consequence of those hard times.

*   *   *

When it came time to choose a college, I was certain of one thing. I wanted to see the wider world, away from Limerick, and away from home. And my parents were wonderful about that. We lived close to the University of Limerick and yet none of us went there. Our parents would have been quite entitled to insist that we did. And yet they didn't. Somehow, they managed to support us all and let us follow the paths we each wanted to follow.

I knew I wanted to go to Dublin, and by then I knew I wanted to study medicine. My parents made that possible. They paid my fees, my accommodation, and put spending money in my bank account every week. At the time, I never thought about how they managed. Now, I think about it a lot.

The six of us were close in age, and at one point four were in college at the same time, and none of us was living at home. My parents didn't have holidays abroad, or nights out. In fact, they had never been out of the country until long after I had left home. Since then, they have travelled the world, I'm glad to say. I still think about their decency and sacrifice, about everything that they went without, in order to let me – all of us – follow our interests. For me, that meant UCD and medicine, and everything that has happened to me since.

CHAPTER TWO
UCD and Emer

I WAS THE ONLY person from my school, the Christian Brothers in Sexton Street, to go to UCD in 1985. I was 18. I may have hardly known anyone, but I did not feel apprehensive. I knew of one of my new classmates, Adrian Moran, indirectly through his brother John, who had been a year ahead of me in school, but otherwise I knew no one. I loved meeting new people and I quickly made new and good friends.

I met Emer Feely, who would become my wife, during the very first week. When I think back, those years in UCD, getting to know Emer and falling in love with her, are deeply inter-twined with the academic experience. Emer was as integral to my time at UCD as anything I learned in lectures.

I remember with great clarity the first time I met her. It was the first week of first year in UCD. Adrian and I went into a lecture together, in the Science building in Belfield. The lecture theatre had steps down from the back on either side, dividing the space into a large middle section and two smaller side sections. Adrian and I sat on the left-hand side behind a small group of people. Right in front of us were two girls, Emer and her friend Martha Ellison, and we just started talking.

I even remember what Emer was wearing – a bright yellow top. And she had a matching bright yellow pen. I think that is why I remember it so clearly. The second day, she wore a pink top and a precisely matching pink pen. I pointed this out to Adrian, saying, 'This is a bit weird . . .' But I was intrigued. A few days later, she came in wearing a tie-dyed blue and white top, and I thought, 'She's hardly going to have a pen to match that.' But she pulled a pen out of her bag, and it was exactly the same colour!

Emer was so glamorous. She had shiny dark hair and long painted nails. She was always beautifully dressed. She was serious, and a good student. Like me, she hadn't come from a medical background. Her father, Frank Feely, was city manager in Dublin for 17 years until 1996. She had three siblings, two older and one younger than her, and all three did electronic engineering, also in UCD. Her older sister Orla is now the first female President of UCD. Emer was always proud of Orla's achievements, and she would have loved to have seen her become President of our alma mater.

Emer grew up on Wainsfort Road in Terenure, very near to where we later lived. She was deeply devoted to her family, and especially close to her mother, Ita. They would talk several times every day, even if it was about nothing more important than *Coronation Street*, of which Ita was a big fan.

Emer and Martha had also been classmates in Our Lady's School in Terenure, where my daughter Clodagh later attended. Martha was full of life. She and Emer were friends almost their entire lives, ever since they met in secondary school. They died within two years of one other, Martha in 2019 and Emer in 2021, both of cancer. Martha was a loyal friend who could be trusted and relied upon in every circumstance. The phrase 'a friend in need is a friend indeed' applied to Martha so well.

She and Emer were always close. She was Emer's 'go-to' person when she was sick. I recall Martha saying how they had both had to stare into the darkness as a consequence of illness and how that gave them an even deeper layer of understanding and connection in their mutual friendship.

Sitting at my kitchen table as I write this book, if I look up I can see a board on my kitchen wall, and pinned to it is Emer's funeral mass booklet. Beside it is Martha's. Whenever I look at the board, it makes me feel sad at just how cruel life was for these two wonderful women who were so full of vitality and fun.

Many of the other people in my pre-med class have remained lifelong friends, particularly Colin Doherty, Eleanor Carey, Barbara Dunne and Emer Henry. Colin is now a Professor of Clinical Neurology and was appointed Head of the Medical School in Trinity in September 2022; a great honour for him and one that we, his close friends, feel part of. Eleanor works with the Health Products Regulatory Authority; Barbara is a consultant pathologist in St James's Hospital; and Emer is a consultant ophthalmologist in Waterford. These were lasting friends in fun times and in hard times.

* * *

Emer made me laugh and I found myself drawn to her from the very beginning. I wasn't in love – yet – but I recall that certainly by the time her debs was to take place, within a few weeks of starting UCD, the four of us – Emer, Martha, Adrian and I – were friendly enough for this to be a topic of conversation. And I know I was interested in the question of who she would be taking.

She invited James Hanley, who lived nearby. James is now one of Ireland's most respected artists and someone I have come to know as a lovely and decent man. In a demonstration of how small Ireland is, James's wife was at school with my sister Breda and his sister Fiona studied psychology at UCD with my sister Aileen. So both Martha and Emer already had partners for the debs. I didn't know how serious Emer and James's relationship was, but at some point soon after the debs, I realised that they were no longer together.

It was a slow-burning thing with me and Emer. We became friends quickly. We went to the Belfield bar together, had lunch, walked around campus, and I began to meet some of her school friends. I remember being introduced to Noeleen, a close friend through primary and secondary school, and taking in the significance of Emer wanting me to meet people who were important to her.

In early February of that first year, I broke my leg playing football. It needed surgery, so I was admitted to St Vincent's Hospital for about ten days. Emer visited me a number of times, as did Emer Henry.

In the next bed to me there was a man from Wicklow, whose name I have forgotten, who had been in a car crash. He was in traction and unable to get out of bed. But his mouth was perfectly alright, and he never stopped talking. He was great company. He was a bit older than me, and forever full of comments, questions and jokes. He called the two Emers 'Big Emer' and 'Little Emer' (my Emer – although she wasn't that yet – was quite tall, almost five foot eleven, and Emer Henry was less so) and he started saying, 'There's something going on there with Big Emer.'

By about April, maybe spurred on by the Wicklow man, I began to think, 'Gosh, I might be a little bit interested here.' As we approached the end of pre-med, I was more and more taken with her. Nothing happened. It was still just a friendship. But we had started to talk on the phone outside college, and I was well aware that something was developing, for me at least.

That did make me feel shyer around her, but our friendship was strong enough that my shyness didn't get in the way. We kept talking, and spending time together, and at one point, as we were coming up to our summer exams, I remember arranging to talk to Martha about this. I thought she could give me a few pointers. She and I met in the Belfield bar, and the first thing I did was to ask for her confidentiality – 'Promise you won't say anything to Emer?' Martha gave her solemn promise . . . and later told me that she couldn't wait to get out of the place to ring Emer. In later years, Martha would tell that story many times, and laugh uproariously.

Martha later married Hugh Mulcahy, a consultant gastroenterologist in St Vincent's Hospital, who became a very important person in our lives. As well as being a good friend, he would later be the person to diagnose Emer. That must have been incredibly hard for him in all the circumstances, especially as at that time Martha was not long recovered from her own initial cancer treatment.

Martha had pledged to go to Lough Derg that summer – she had bartered a pilgrimage for exam results. She thought she hadn't done enough study for one of the exams – I think it was physics – and so she traded with God: 'I'll go to Lough Derg and you have to let me pass my exams.' She did pass, and Emer went with her – they did so much together. While they were there, they met my aunt, my mother's youngest sister, Anne, who worked in Nenagh hospital. When I heard Anne would be going to Lough Derg on the same trip, I wrote a letter to Emer; and I asked Anne to look out for two young women from Dublin, one tall and dark, the other smaller and blonde. The letter was delivered. Emer wrote to me, telling me this. I don't remember much of the detail of what she said, but I can remember she wrote back, and the way that felt like something significant.

That summer, I had a job in a hotel in Limerick. But I badly wanted to get back to Dublin. I travelled up and down to Dublin as often as I could over the course of the summer to go to parties and nights out organised by college friends. But my main focus was to see Emer. Most of the time, I was nervous and lacked confidence. I was so besotted with Emer that I was afraid to make a move. Somehow, I thought it was better to wait for the 'perfect time' rather than to make a clumsy move and mess things up for ever!

By the time we came back to college for the start of second year, I could hardly think about anything other than how I could find a way. I recall the pressure very clearly – and I was letting the pressure build up. I was 'class rep' that year, and the most important function of class rep is to organise the class parties. Which I did. These were meticulously planned: organising venues, hiring music systems, issuing tickets and so on. We used to get free beer kegs from the main alcohol companies, which had student representatives in UCD. At the time, I thought that was great. Now, I have a very different view of that form of promotion.

Colin designed magnificent posters for us that we printed and displayed around UCD and the clinical teaching sites. Colin's artistic talent comes from his mother, Patricia Hurl, a great Irish expressionist painter, who had a wonderful retrospective at IMMA in February 2023.

I remember the anticipation I felt in advance of these nights out and wondering if tonight would be the night. Sure enough, the night we got together for the first time was at a second year class party in Newman House that I had organised. All the work and planning had paid off. I can still hear Berlin's

'Take My Breath Away'. Every time I hear that song it stops me in my tracks and brings me back to 6 November 1986.

Throughout the remainder of second year in college, our relationship evolved slowly, centring on weekends and class nights out. On one early date, which still makes me cringe, I invited Emer to my flat and really set out to impress her with the fanciest recipe I could come up with. Roast chicken and roast potatoes. I cook a lot nowadays, but that was probably my first attempt at a proper roast. Somehow, she stayed with me.

During third year, Emer started to come to our house in Limerick on a regular basis – a weekend at Christmas, at New Year, a few days in the summer holidays – meeting my parents and my sisters.

My sisters and I were chatting recently, reminiscing about those times. Sinead, the second youngest, remembers Christmas 1987. She was almost 15 at the time, and Aoife, the youngest, 13. With so many girls, there was always activity and noise in our house. A dispute arose between Sinead and Aoife. Sinead remembers that Emer intervened to restore peace. Clearly my sisters felt comfortable enough to be themselves and have a row in front of Emer, and just as clearly she felt able to intervene. These were the beginnings of enduring and close friendships between Emer and each of my sisters.

I don't ever remember asking Emer, 'Would you like to go out with me?' It was just a point we arrived at. And it was the same with our engagement when that came: it wasn't a bended knee moment with an engagement ring. It was a gradual evolution, a knowing, that we came to together. From the age of 19 it was clear to me that Emer was the person I wanted to be with.

* * *

Emer was a wonderful person, full of love, kindness and care. She was the life and soul of every gathering of family or friends. While she could be shy and reserved, that was only to those who didn't know her. Once Clodagh and Ronan were born they became the centre of her world. Every waking moment and a few sleeping ones were about them; they could not have hoped for a better mother.

In 2016, when Emer was quite unwell, I had the idea of asking the people in her life to write or share something about who Emer was to them and what she meant to them. I often found it sad to hear people being spoken of in glowing terms after they had died and that they didn't get to hear these lovely personal tributes from the people in their lives. I wanted Emer to hear what others thought of her.

Family, friends, college contemporaries, workmates and school friends were included. The contributions were made into a soft leather-bound book with copies for Clodagh and Ronan. I was not sure how Emer would feel about it when we gave it to her as a Christmas present in 2016, but she loved it. Many times over the following years she would take it from the shelf to leaf through it.

What came through in what everyone said of her was her wicked sense of humour. How quick-witted she was. How loyal and loving she was. And how evident to everyone her selfless love for Clodagh and Ronan was.

CHAPTER THREE

UCD and After

1985–1991

MEDICINE IN UCD BEGAN with pre-med, which was quite similar to the first year science course. It was the only year we spent in Belfield. After that we moved to Earlsfort Terrace for almost three years for pre-clinical tuition-based learning, and then on to almost full-time hospital-based experience for the last two years. We didn't see a patient or a ward until after Easter in the fourth year. Trying to connect what we learned in lectures to the relevance of what we would have to do as doctors with real patients could be difficult. I remember feeling that, after more than three years in medical school, I was no further down the road of understanding what life was going to be like as a doctor than I had been when I left school. I found that unsettling.

The exciting part of medical training for me began when we entered the hospital for the residence – 'res' – year. For my res year I attended St Vincent's Hospital. I loved it right from the start. Being in the hospital, being involved in clinical inter- actions, learning in that kind of environment – everything clicked into place and made sense. I loved the buzz of it. I would hang around in the evenings and do extra hours in the hospital, especially in the emergency department.

As part of that res year, we were attached to consultant-led teams for successive two-week or longer periods. We covered seven or eight different teams across medicine and surgery and therefore interacted with many of the consultants and the senior nursing staff. It was very hierarchical. Some of the consultants were very detached figures, but others were wonderful hands-on teachers, really engaged and clearly enthusiastic about teaching students at the bedside. A ward round with the consultant could be almost ceremonial. It would involve fifteen or so people, all more important than you. You knew very well where your place was – to stay out of trouble, and get the right answers to questions that would be randomly fired at you. It was a great time of discovery and enjoyment. There we were, wearing white coats, in the wards and walking around. A lot of patients don't make a distinction. If you're in a white coat, as far as they're concerned you're a doctor. They will talk to you, ask you questions, listen carefully to your answers.

Surgery was what interested me most. It was hard not to be captivated by the bright lights and urgency of the operating theatre; the heady potential to save or change someone's life. I remember late one night being involved, in a small way, in a liver transplant. People were needed to bring blood from the blood bank in the hospital to the operating theatre, and a few of us medical students were asked to volunteer. That was exciting. Liver transplants were right at the cutting edge of technical developments at the time, and St Vincent's was the only hospital in Ireland where they were happening.

Everything started to feel tangible. For years, it felt like we had been learning science subjects rather than clinical subjects. When I found myself in the real-life setting of a patient's bedside, I learned to join up the physiology or the pathology with the biochemistry or the pharmacology, and bring it all together to problem-solve real clinical issues and questions. It all made sense in that way and I found this method much easier to understand, absorb and learn.

There were times when I was involved in consultations when a patient was being given bad news. Sometimes someone would receive important, life-changing news, with no other relatives present, but 15 people – a full medical team – standing around a bed. Considering that now, and with everything I have learned and experienced since, it is clear to me that that is not appropriate. I would stop short of saying that doesn't happen now, but I would like to think it doesn't happen as much as it used to.

*   *   *

One of the things we were learning as medical students, very gradually, was to have confidence in our own abilities and decisions. There was an emphasis on the importance of being decisive, sometimes with imperfect or incomplete information, and on the need to make the best decision at a point in time, as opposed to the perfect decision. A lot of training is implicitly focused on that. This requirement also demands personal skills and attributes; some people are naturally good at it and some people struggle. As a doctor, you learn the importance of believing in yourself. In a large teaching hospital, this happens quite gradually; you might be called upon during the on-call period to make an assessment of a patient who is unwell, for example. In smaller hospitals, the level of responsibility taken by more junior doctors can be greater.

I only understood how cosseted we were as interns in St Vincent's Hospital when I entered my GP training programme. The change was head-spinning. One day I was one intern among many in a large teaching hospital, and literally the next day I was the senior house officer (SHO) in paediatrics in

Limerick, starting with three months of neonatology. As a neonatology SHO, I was the only person from the paediatric team in the hospital at night. That was daunting. The majority of babies are born perfectly healthy, but some can be really sick. Limerick has a large maternity unit and sick babies were a common enough occurrence.

Many high-risk pregnancies are diagnosed prenatally – a woman might have a history that flags a risk, or perhaps it is twin or multiple pregnancy or there are signs indicating possible foetal distress. I was on standby for these and for any assisted delivery, meaning forceps, suction or caesarean section. Once the baby emerges, he or she is given to you to make an assessment. The initial assessments in the minutes, sometimes seconds, after birth are critically important. If the baby is born 'flat' – where there is no sound, no response – that is very scary. You can't get it wrong.

I was 25, still quite young, and that is a huge level of responsibility and very different from being an intern in a large teaching hospital. Initially it was intense, but I adapted fairly quickly. If you spend all your time thinking of the things that could go wrong, you would be too inhibited to function.

One memory stands out from that time: I was called to be present at the delivery of a baby in the middle of the night. The mum had had an epidural anaesthetic and needed instrumental help to deliver the baby. She had been in labour for a while. The midwives were there and the obstetric consultant (the mother was a private patient) was preparing to carry out the delivery. The patient's partner was sitting on the stool next to her. When the baby came out he was handed to me and I examined him under the lamp. Everything was perfectly normal. While I was counting the fingers and toes, the man who had been sitting on the stool next to the mother came over. I turned to him and said 'Congratulations', to which he responded, 'I'm the f***ing anaesthetist'. Even the exhausted mum had a good laugh at me!

*   *   *

The GP training scheme was, at the time, a three-year programme (it is now four), made up of two years of relevant hospital jobs and one year as a GP registrar in a training practice. You work as a doctor and are paid, but you are still in training. The two years in hospital were usually broken into four six-month postings covering obstetrics, paediatrics, medicine, psychiatry and some other areas. In Limerick we had an opportunity to have one six-month period in which half was devoted to ENT (ear, nose and throat surgery) and half as a community-based medical officer running child development assessment and vaccination clinics. Each of these was very valuable for general practice training. ENT problems are a very big component of general practice. Furthermore, you get to see plenty of healthy children in developmental and vaccination clinics. This reminds you that most children are, thankfully, healthy. Something that is worth remembering as a GP when you have worked in a paediatric hospital position.

I finished my GP training in Athea, in west Limerick, on the border with Kerry, with a wonderful GP, Kieran Murphy, who only recently retired. Being a GP is a calling in itself, and rural general practice is a particularly vocational undertaking. Kieran was described by one of our tutors as the type who would have liked to take all his patients home in the back of his car and mind them. That captured him well. His patients loved him and he was very dedicated to their wellbeing.

That year with Kieran was very formative for me and fed into my growing awakening and understanding about the relationship between health and wellbeing, and how the two are deeply interconnected. Athea is a small rural community, and I came across examples of rural deprivation that I wouldn't have thought existed. Naively, I had an unconscious bias that poverty and deprivation belonged to urban settings. I was wrong. Working as a rural GP, you see it laid bare. I recall people living in mobile homes with no running water; men living alone in houses with no electricity. The kind of thing I had no idea existed in Ireland. In general practice, you get to see people in their homes and to observe the social circumstances some people have to live in and endure. It was a profound experience.

Something I found difficult was the reality that, as a GP working in the community in which you also live, which is usually the case for rural general practice, privacy is a challenge. The people of Athea were lovely, and I don't mean to suggest this was anything to do with them. Perhaps I found it more difficult because I did not grow up in a rural setting.

Living in the community as a doctor brings other challenges. A woman presented to me one day with symptoms and signs of depression. In the consultation it emerged that her partner, who I knew socially, was physically abusive to her. I found that very difficult.

But I knew I wouldn't be staying in Athea. I would have to pass the Irish College of General Practitioners exams in the coming summer; Emer and I were engaged and looking forward to getting married the following summer, 1995. She was also training as a GP, in a practice in Ballyfermot which she loved, and I was travelling to Dublin to see her every weekend I was not on call.

I knew that my professional interest was elsewhere than general practice. I had a strong and growing interest in public health, and by the time I had finished in Athea I had already applied to return to UCD to complete a master's degree in public health.

*   *   *

There is often immediate gratification in clinical medicine. It is the connection between interacting with a patient, listening, making decisions and, hopefully, achieving a speedy and good outcome for them. There is almost immediate feedback and response to the choices you make as a practitioner. In that way, it is very different from public health, the area I subsequently chose to specialise in, where there isn't anything like that real-time impact; the effect of individual decisions is harder to trace and outcomes unfold over many years.

There were various moments during my years of study and training that focused my interest on public health. One of these was a surgical elective I did in Nenagh hospital during my last summer in college. An elective was something you organised on your own initiative, outside the standard course. I chose this because I was interested in surgery, and I picked Nenagh because my aunt was head of catering there. I knew that in a small hospital I might get more hands-on experience. And I did. As the only medical student in the hospital, I was some-thing of a novelty for the other doctors, who gave me plenty of their time and tuition.

A consultant surgeon, Mr David McAvinchy, asked me to do a review of evidence related to appendicitis. What concerned him was how many people who went to surgery with a diagnosis of appendicitis turned out in fact to have a normal appendix. Once they got as far as the operating table, the appendix was removed whether it was diseased or not. But it meant that a person who did not have appendicitis had an unnecessary general anaesthetic and operation. Mr McAvinchy wondered what tests could be used to improve the certainty of the diagnosis prior to surgery. He had me look at published research studies relating to a variety of tests as to their performance characteristics and how effective they were. Examining the literature about various tests (blood tests, ultrasound, X-rays and clinical signs), I tried to make assessments of their predictive value, sensitivity and specificity in appendicitis. This might send most people to sleep, but I loved the mathematics of it. This is clinical epidemiology, and learning about it really opened my mind.

Even though he didn't express it in these terms, David McAvinchy was teaching me how to think. It was my 'eureka' moment. And I have him to thank for it. I remember coming back to college for our final medical year after that elective and telling my classmates what I'd been doing. I'm sure they were bored stiff! But through that experience, and the thinking behind it, I was switched on to the idea of epidemiology and public health. Intellectually and in every other way, it appealed to me.

The more I learned, the more I found myself thinking about causes and consequences of illness. About how you can treat an infection of some kind with an antibiotic, but you may not be treating the underlying cause. And how, if you don't treat that underlying cause, there will always be more instances of the illness. If you keep having to help people out of a river, at a certain point are you not compelled to walk upstream and ask, Why are all these people ending up in the water? I became more interested in that kind of question. And in wondering how I might be able to do something to influence these causes. I didn't want to end up in a career in which I was dealing only with the end results of social inequality, poverty and lack of opportunity; all things that contribute to disease. I wanted to walk further upstream. To see if I could do something about these causes.

I became passionately interested in public health as a way to influence policy, to effect change to the determinants of disease.

* * *

Once I had left Athea at the end of June, I worked as a locum GP in Balbriggan, County Dublin, throughout that gloriously sunny summer of 1995. Emer and I were married on 19 August in her local church, St Pius X in Terenure. We celebrated our wedding with 120 family and close friends in Barberstown Castle in Straffan, County Kildare. We took three weeks off for our honeymoon on Paradise Island in the Bahamas. In late September I enrolled on the master's degree in public health programme in UCD. I was a full-time student again and Emer was the breadwinner. The following year, we swapped those roles – Emer went back to college and did that same master's, and I worked.

I loved that extra year in UCD. I found the topics fascinating, and everything I learned made sense. That programme taught me to think in a very different way. As a doctor, you're taught to think about the patient in front of you, and everything to do with the patient in front of you, particularly how to maximise the benefit and outcome. And that is right and proper. The master's in public health taught me to look in a different way at health issues and diseases I was already familiar with. We explored the best way of responding, at a population level, to a given disease. Is it by improving hospital services? Not necessarily. Sometimes intervention needs to start far earlier. You have to find ways to intervene on the disease course long before it reaches a hospital setting.

Diabetes is a good illustration of the difference I found between clinical and public health approaches to the same illness. As a GP or clinical doctor, I was taught to think about the individual diabetic patient – how to improve their compliance with exercise or medication, how to enhance control of their blood sugar and how to slow down the emergence of any complications of their diseases. In the master's programme, I was now learning to frame the problem of diabetes in a population context: How do we prevent its risk factors? How do we detect the disease early? Should we screen for it? How should we organise services to provide better prevention and treatment? How do we empower patients to take better control of their illness? The public health aim, I now understood, is to improve the whole population's experience of diabetes, while accepting that you won't prevent or improve every single case, and to evaluate the performance of all services and the whole population's experience on that basis.

The very intangibility of prevention and public health can make for a hard sell. It can be difficult to get public and political support and attention. 'Man does not get cancer' is never a headline. One of our master's lecturers phrased the challenge perfectly: 'No one ever thanks you for not having cholera.' We don't have cholera in this country: not because we have hospital-based services that treat cholera; but because we prevent it through hygiene and sanitation and a proper understanding of its cause.

This way of thinking was a revelation for me. I had found my pathway. Public health became my vocation.

CHAPTER FOUR
A Hard Lesson Learned

As MEDICAL STUDENTS IN the late 1980s, we were not taught in any detail about patient safety. In fact, patient safety did not emerge as a clear and distinct health policy issue until the early 2000s (a key milestone was *To Err is Human*, published by the Institute of Medicine in the USA in 2000). I became quite involved in patient safety over a long period of time in my role as Chief Medical Officer (CMO). But my own personal awakening to its importance stems from an incident that occurred during my time as an intern. Something happened that had the power to have changed the entire course of my life.

First, what is patient safety? It is a branch of health policy and health service practice that is concerned with ensuring that health services are safe. A safe system is one in which the risk of something going wrong is minimised; in which the chance of picking up something that goes wrong is maximised; in which there are effective systems to investigate and derive learning from errors when they do occur; in which measures are put in place to apply those lessons; and in which monitoring takes place to ensure the implementation of those lessons. That is a safe system. One that is open, self-questioning, continuously learning and improving.

So what happened to me to make this really stick in my mind? I was well into the second six months of my internship in St Vincent's. The first six months was as a medical intern and now I was a surgical intern. Each night there were four interns on call. As one of the two on-call interns in surgery, I would be busy in the evenings and would share the workload on the surgical wards with the other surgical intern. The pair of medical interns had their own workload with medical wards. The other surgical intern and I would split the night from midnight to eight in the morning; one in bed for the first four hours, and the other for the second four hours. That way, hopefully, you would get at least four hours' sleep.

One night I was walking back to the residence after completing a call to a surgical ward. I took a shortcut through one of the medical wards and passed by the nurses' station. I stopped to say hello. Having been a medical intern previously, I knew the nurses there. They asked if I would do them a favour: would I give a first dose of an intravenous antibiotic to a patient? They couldn't get hold of the medical intern who should be doing it, she wasn't answering her pager. They named the person. I had by then had enough experience to know that some people might be nice or be great craic, but weren't that great to be on call with!

Where an intravenous antibiotic has been prescribed, the first dose must be given by a doctor in case there is a significant allergic reaction. You have to put in an intravenous line, draw the antibiotic up, mix it, administer it and so on. It is a time-consuming process. Right then, in the middle of the night, when I was on my way back to the residence, I didn't want to have to do this. It was someone else's job, and that someone was probably in bed, asleep. Bed was where I wanted to be. But the nurses persuaded me. They said the patient – a woman – needed the antibiotic, and they had already done most of the preparation, making it much quicker for me to carry out. They had drawn up the dose, she had a central line in place and so I would not need to insert one. Everything was ready to go. I was very tired but I agreed to do it.

I took everything they gave me, went into the patient, introduced myself, explained what I was there to do, and I began injecting the antibiotic into the central line. Only then did I say, 'By the way, are you allergic to anything?'

'Yes,' she said. 'I am. Penicillin.'

Penicillin was what I was injecting her with. I felt like I had been hit over the head. I had half a syringe administered to a patient and now she was telling me she had an allergy to penicillin.

The risk was an immediate and life-threatening allergic reaction to penicillin, with swelling and constriction of airways. In this case, the patient seemed fine. So far. I immediately stopped injecting. Only about a third of the dose had gone in. I removed the syringe and stayed with her long enough to be sure she wasn't having an immediate reaction. I quickly checked her medical chart – sure enough, it was documented: 'allergic to penicillin.' I called the registrar on-call in a state of controlled panic. I told him what had happened. By now 10 minutes had elapsed.

'How is she now?' he asked.

'She seems fine,' I replied

He gave a knowing laugh and said, 'She is not allergic to penicillin at all!'

I had unintentionally tested her allergy, and it turned out she didn't have one. I know now there are many people who say they are allergic to penicillin, but when you question them about what that means, they might say, 'I got Augmentin once and I vomited.' That is not an allergy. Thankfully, this patient was in that category.

I was incredibly lucky.

But that was a dramatic learning. I learned that in order for one thing to go very wrong, you often need many little things to happen or not happen as they should. And that this can arise even when everyone involved is trying to do their best. This woman wasn't my patient. I wasn't the medical intern on call. I was half-asleep. The nurses were encouraging me, and telling me the work was all done; the woman had a central line in. All the steps I would go through if I was properly assessing the patient myself, I was being told had been done already. I was being encouraged and agreed to do a favour. I did the favour, and there were very nearly terrible consequences. Obviously the most serious of these would have been for the patient. She could have died. My first sense of relief was naturally for her. But the consequences for me would have been considerable too.

I was the doctor; the responsibility would have rested with me, regardless of the circumstances. I did not check for myself whether this person was allergic, and that was my failing, no matter how it came about. But mine wasn't the only failing. How did a person who was apparently allergic to penicillin ever have Augmentin prescribed to them? Prescribing and dispensing errors are common. Systems to minimise these are not as widespread as they should be.

When I look back now, I know that incident was not investigated afterwards in the way it would or should be investigated if such an event were to happen nowadays. The opportunity to learn a lesson from such a near-miss so as to reduce the risk of a recurrence was not taken. But the lesson stayed with me.

* * *

That gave me an early interest in patient safety and how public health thinking should be applied to addressing it. I've come to understand that improving patient safety requires many layers of protection, so that something like my experience is much less likely to happen. There is a growing understanding that doing things systematically, learning and applying lessons, will make the experience of healthcare safer.

Change is more urgent than many people might expect. The rate of iatrogenic – meaning doctor- or health service-induced – illness or harm is surprisingly high. This could mean, for example, an infection picked up in hospital, a prescribing error, an error in a diagnosis, a misread scan or an incorrect surgical procedure.

A 2016 study published in the *British Medical Journal* found that in the United States, medical errors are the third leading cause of death, after heart disease and cancer. It estimated that medical errors may contribute to more than 250,000 deaths annually. Other studies suggest that medical harm is more widespread than mortality statistics suggest. A 2018 study published in the journal *Health Affairs* estimated that one in ten patients experience harm while receiving medical care, much of which is preventable.

It is important to make clear that a system that is safe is not a system in which no harm occurs, and in which adverse outcomes are always avoided. The reality is that delivery of healthcare is a risky business – risk cannot be fully eliminated. Patients are sick and vulnerable; services are imperfect; the science and technologies are imperfect. And the doctors, nurses and other professionals, despite being highly trained, are not perfect. Things will go wrong. A service that does not accept that cannot be considered safe.

So much of patient safety comes down to communication; the interfaces between people. That is where many things go right or wrong – the transfer of information from the brain of one doctor or nurse to another, such that the patient has full and proper continuity of care, as responsibility is transferred from one health professional to the next.

There is really only one opportunity to maintain trust and confidence on the part of a patient who has been harmed and possibly traumatised. That is right at the start when something is believed to have gone wrong. It requires open, clear and effective dialogue. That may be a very difficult conversation to have, but it is critical to establishing and maintaining patients' trust and confidence, which in turn are important determinants of good outcomes. There is evidence that in systems where that happens there is much less likelihood of care breaking down – which is the most important thing – but also far less likelihood of litigation.

Other industries have implemented means of reducing the risks of communication errors. The airline industry is a good example. Following a devastating crash in Las Palmas in the late 1970s, that sector began to understand that clear and good communication, checklists for all common tasks and an open, blame-free reporting culture were integral to making flying as safe as it could be.

Healthcare is more complex, many will say in response. And it is. But it nonetheless has much to learn from these changes in culture and from the standardisation of information and communication. There is still quite a way to go to make healthcare as safe as it can be.

That night in St Vincent's the incident was, thankfully, a near miss, but that woman could have died. It was just luck that she didn't. I remember thinking how close I had come to disaster. There was nothing in what I did that intended harm, and yet I did something that could have caused great harm to her.

CHAPTER FIVE
Early Married Life

THE DAY WE CAME back from our honeymoon, I found Emer in tears in the sitting room of our new apartment. I wondered if it was that she was sorry to be back. But she was homesick. This was the first time Emer had ever lived away from her family, and she missed them, her mother in particular. Although I could understand, I couldn't fully relate to how she felt. After all, I had left home aged 18, ten years earlier, and with a sense of excitement. Her reaction was touchingly true to what I knew of her – and what I learned even more deeply over the following years together. Her love of family was profound. Her sense of home, of place, of loyalty to the people she loved, was the central thing for her.

Of course Emer got over her homesickness, and we were very happy in Milltown for three years, before buying our first house, a new-build in Castleknock. And it wasn't long before we were lucky enough to start our own family. Clodagh was born on 10 January 2001 while we were in Castleknock.

At this stage, I had finished the master's in UCD, and was close to completing the four-year training programme in public health. Usually six people are recruited to this training programme every year. It runs much like the training programmes in all other medical specialisms. You become a specialist registrar and rotate in a planned way through a number of different positions over the four years. When I joined the programme in 1997, I had competed successfully to be trained in the Eastern region, i.e. Dublin. Shortly afterwards, the training programme was amended to make it one national programme, whereas prior to that each regional health board had its own position. After two years in the Eastern Health Board in Dublin, I was assigned to the Midland Health Board, based in Tullamore, for one year.

At the time I was unhappy with that imposed change. Emer and I had just bought a new house in Dublin and now we would have the added expense of me having to commute and to find mid-week accommodation elsewhere. Later, however, I came to see this as a valuable and interesting broadening of horizons.

Emer entered the public health training programme in 1999, two years after me, and her initial assignment was in Limerick City, away from our new home in Castleknock. It began at the same time as my one-year assignment to Tullamore. We rented a flat in Nenagh, which gave us equal commuting time – an hour each way. From Monday to Thursday, Emer would drive to and from Limerick, I would drive to and from Tullamore, and every Friday we'd come back home to Dublin.

When I finished my year in Tullamore in July 2000, I was assigned to the Office of the Chief Medical Officer, Dr Jim Kiely, in the Department of Health. I was back in Dublin. Emer had one more year's assignment to complete in Limerick. She moved in with my sister Breda, who lives in Raheen in Limerick City with her husband, Tom Considine. By then, Breda had two young children, Brian and Emma. She and Emer had always been very close. Living together, they became closer still. Emer also always had a close relationship with Brian and Emma from that time. By then Emer was pregnant with Clodagh, and I found great comfort, as she was getting more advanced in her pregnancy, in knowing that she was going home to Breda and Tom every evening.

That was an unsettled time in our lives. There was a lot of moving around, and a lot of time apart. I can remember Friday evenings, tensely waiting for Emer to drive back to Dublin, especially in the later stages of her pregnancy. But once Clodagh was born, that was the end of the out-of-Dublin part of her training, and when Emer resumed the training programme after her maternity leave in July 2001, she was assigned to the Office of the Chief Medical Officer. I had just been appointed on a temporary contract as deputy CMO. Now Emer would be in the office next door for six months!

When we had Clodagh and Ronan, Emer always wanted to be with them. To do things with them and for them. Everything, for Emer, was about the children. Once Clodagh and Ronan started school, she chose to only work mornings. I know we were lucky, and privileged – both financially, and in terms of having a career that enabled her to do that. Working part-time is not a choice that is available to many people.

*   *   *

Emer was particularly motivated by environmental health issues, hospital bed occupancy and the question of palliative care. As part of her training programme, while we lived in Nenagh, Emer was involved in a large project at Silvermines, County Tipperary, where there was a tailings pond. These are areas into which waterborne waste mining tailings are pumped, allowing the sedimentation (separation) of solids from water. The pond is generally impounded with a dam. A high lead content was found in soil, water and grass there, and autopsies on a number of cattle found high lead levels in the carcasses. That meant potential human contamination, and questions arose about the potential chronic effects on health. The local community was rightly very concerned. Chronic build-up of lead can have long-term effects, especially developmentally and intellectually, on children.

Studies needed to be done to establish the facts, and engagement needed to be undertaken with the local community. Emer was part of the team carrying out this work. She was effectively the lead investigator, and she did some really ground-breaking work, such that Kevin Kelleher, director of public health for the region, was really generous in his praise for her. I remember going with her one night to a community meeting in Silvermines. I sat at the back of the hall, which was full of genuinely concerned people. All the local politicians were there. It was a difficult meeting and Emer was right there, with her hand fully in the wound, as it were. I could see how good she was at her work, at generating trust on the part of the local community and at explaining things in difficult circumstances. I felt so much pride watching her, seeing her in her element; capable and reassuring. That study was ultimately written up by Emer and her colleagues and published in the *Irish Medical Journal*.

The other area that moved her was, ironically as it later turned out, palliative care. The completion of specialist training in public health requires a Membership examination. The first part of the exam is written; the second part requires a detailed piece of research written up as a thesis. Emer chose to survey population needs for in-patient palliative care, as part of the case being made to fund the development of Blackrock Hospice. There was no hospice at the time in that part of Dublin. Noel Smyth, solicitor to Ben Dunne, and his wife provided funding, and Emer played a pivotal role. The Blackrock Hospice is part of her legacy.

What interested Emer was place of death, and the extent to which choice is or can be taken into account. The Irish Hospice

Foundation published research in 2021 which shows that 40 per cent of all deaths take place in hospital, 23 per cent at home and 8 per cent in a hospice. An acute hospital environment is not where most people would choose to die. Sometimes this can't be avoided, but often it could be. The development of services so that people can have better and more informed choices is something Emer strongly believed in. No one wants to die, but we will all face death at some point. There are steps that can be taken to make this a better experience, not just for the person, but for those around them.

The irony of course is that, later, Emer found herself using these very services.

* * *

After her training, Emer was appointed as a specialist in public health in the HSE, in Dr Steevens' Hospital, opposite Heuston Station. She worked in a very hands-on way in infectious disease control and other aspects of public health in Dublin and the eastern region.

The pandemic has highlighted the role of public health doctors and brought more public understanding to the role they play. In public health departments, they work in teams with other professionals; infection control nurses, environmental health officers, surveillance scientists and others. The tools of their trade, which we all saw during the course of the pandemic, include transmission control, contact tracing, case management, surveillance and reporting, as well as communication. Their work includes investigating incidents and outbreaks of infectious disease; monitoring and reporting on community health and health inequalities; health promotion; and disease prevention. It also includes service developments that offer further protection and resilience for health services.

Emer was a member of the National Emergency Department Task Force in its early years in the mid-2000s. She was the driving force behind a national study, using a standardised and validated tool, of appropriateness of hospital admission. During the conduct of that study she visited every hospital in the country. That work showed that a very high proportion of people in hospital beds at any point in time did not have a medical need to be there. They could and should be cared for either in other settings or as outpatient attendees. That fact will not surprise anyone, perhaps, but Emer's work showed the number was approximately one-third of people nationally and, in the case of some hospitals, well in excess of half.

That work should be replicated on a continuing basis. It provided an evidential basis as to why we need to think more in terms of better models and pathways of care rather than simply building additional in-patient beds. The pandemic demonstrated clearly the risks of picking up infection in hospitals, which underscores the importance of aiming to ensure we only have people in a hospital bed if their requirement for medical care is such that they cannot be cared for elsewhere. The work that Emer led provided a very important baseline which could be regularly monitored to measure progress in integrated models of care for patients who are less hospital bed-dependent.

Emer continued to work at Dr Steevens' for a long time after she was diagnosed and was supported enormously by her colleagues. There was a time when she would drive into St James's Hospital for chemotherapy, then on to Dr Steevens' for work. She wanted to keep working for as long as possible, and she wanted to continue taking on interesting and challenging projects. This was important for her sense of normality.

* * *

Clodagh's arrival caused great excitement in Emer's family. She was the first grandchild on the Feely side. Emer's parents and siblings were so enthusiastic about babysitting that we would get regular, eager phone calls – 'Are you going out tonight?' Emer loved going to the cinema, and so that is what we did. I think we must have seen every movie that was released over a period of about two years.

When Clodagh was a young toddler, we decided to move from Castleknock to Terenure, to be close to her parents and the community in which Emer had grown up. Not only did that bring us closer to the source of baby-sitting, it also made Emer happy to be within easy walking distance of Frank and Ita as they were getting older. We moved in the summer of 2002, not long before Ronan was born.

Emer's six-month attachment to the Department of Health was her first six months at work after Clodagh was born. She was based in Hawkins House, near City Quay, a building that has since been torn down, and not before time. Emer and I used to joke that the best thing about working in it was you couldn't see it on the cityscape. Then Minister for Health Mary Harney's well-known verdict on it was 'Half the windows don't open and the other half don't close!'

Working and having small children is very intense. I still remember how hard it was, particularly at the start. There was a 5.15pm train every day from Connolly Station to Castleknock. The next train after that was at 6.20pm, so it was a hard deadline every day to ensure we were on time to collect Clodagh from her childminder. I still remember the stress of clock-watching, running across the river to Connolly Station. Tens of thousands of families are doing that very same thing every day; running to collect children, under constant pressure. It is not easy. Looked at from a wider perspective, this raises many big questions – about childcare, transportation, sustainability and climate change. We need to talk far more about our well-being as a society when we discuss these issues. They are not solely economic questions. Anybody who has had children in childcare has lived those kinds of struggles, and battles; the arguments around 'I did it three times last week, it's your turn today.' And even though I would like to recall it as more equal, in truth I think Emer was running that race to the train much more often than I was. I know she found it hard to leave Clodagh when she was so young. We had to adapt, as everyone does. And we did, but the challenges of that time have stayed with me.

I remember the constant worry, too: 'Are they okay? Does that temperature mean anything? Do they seem out of sorts?' I don't think medical training helps very much with that. There were times it was handy, but there were times when it was quite the opposite. As a parent who is a doctor, you generally either under-react or over-react, and at different times I've done both. You end up making medical assessments of your own children, which is never a good idea. That is the kind of responsibility that needs to be somebody else's.

Both Clodagh and Ronan, as toddlers, had occasional mild bronchiolitis, which produces a wheeze; and they had inhalers for short periods of time. Happily, they have both grown out of it completely, but there was a day when Clodagh had a bad chest infection, and I remember speeding to Our Lady's Hospital for Sick Children, Crumlin, seriously worried. Within a couple of hours it was thankfully obvious that everything was okay. I knew I had totally overreacted. And I knew why.

The truth is, your judgement is completely clouded by the relationship. You can't make any kind of objective assessment. Instead, possibly the most useful thing to ask yourself is, 'What would I do if someone else came to me? Am I the best person to make this decision? Is my mind sufficiently clear and objective to enable me to make the right assessment and the right decision?' These are all questions that had later relevance in the context of Emer's diagnosis.

You need to take yourself out of the situation. Stop being the doctor and be the dad. Or the husband. I don't always follow that advice, but I try to because I believe in the value of it.

CHAPTER SIX
Deputy Chief Medical Officer
2001–2008

I WAS APPOINTED DEPUTY CMO on a temporary contract in early 2001. As soon as the CMO, Dr Jim Kiely, asked me to consider it, I jumped at the chance. Since my days as a medical student, I had become increasingly drawn to health policy. I am still immensely grateful to Jim for having enough faith in me at that stage in my career.

At the time, immediately before Christmas 2000, I was coming to the end of the four-year public health training programme. I had interviewed for and been offered a permanent job in the newly established National Disease Surveillance Centre (NDSC). The NDSC later became the Health Protection Surveillance Centre (HPSC), which played a prominent and very effective role in the pandemic. I turned down the permanent NDSC job to take a temporary one in the Department of Health. Emer was somewhat worried about what her dad, Frank, would say. Emer's family visited us that Christmas and we discussed the decision I had to make. Fortunately, I had not only Emer's full support but her family's too. That was important, especially as this was a few weeks before Clodagh was born. About a year later, the permanent position came up and I went through the process of applying, interviewing, and being offered the job on a permanent basis.

* * *

During my first years as deputy CMO, I was very involved with the primary care strategy *Primary Care: A New Direction* (published in 2001). Having come from general practice training, this was an area of personal interest for me. I knew there was a considerable need for more emphasis on primary care. The concept of the primary care strategy was to join up all the pieces that already existed in the community – GP, public health nurse, physiotherapy, occupational therapy, social work and so on – into a single primary care team. The focus of each team would be to serve the same population, thereby delivering a greater quality and extent of care.

Without integration of services, you miss vital opportunities such as better emphasis on disease prevention, better care within the community and better chronic disease management. The premise of the primary care strategy was that if we could provide more of this generalist foundation-level care, we might help to anticipate and prevent issues, and manage them before they required more specialised hospital-based services.

Working on that strategy taught me a valuable lesson. I was a brand-new deputy CMO, enthusiastically involved in a project that I could see a clear need for. I had opportunities to talk about it to the Minister for Health, Micheál Martin, and he was very supportive. We had lift-off. Or so it seemed.

In fact, that is just the beginning. Once a policy has been approved by government, it must be followed through, and funded. There needed to be engagement with unions and other stakeholder interests. There needed to be more staff, more team-building and more IT systems to enable people to integrate their work. And there needed to be significant investment in capital infrastructure.

Not all the recommended improvements happened. At least not to the extent we had hoped, or to the extent needed. My close colleague Fergal Goodman and I had a path worn over and back to the Department of Finance, making a case for capital allowances to support the development of primary care centres where a team could be shown to be needed and present. I think we made a compelling case. But we got little change out of the officials in the Department of Finance.

It may be difficult for some to see health expenditure as an investment rather than a cost, a drain on resources and a brake on national economic competitiveness. I believe a more modern view of health expenditure is needed as investment in health and investment in people. Ultimately that means viewing the economy as being there to serve our wellbeing as human beings and not the other way around. That will take time. And it will take confidence in the HSE and the Department of Health on the part of those finance and public expenditure officials.

Over the course of my professional career, that was one of the more disappointing things I have been involved with. To see the limited progress on meaningful developments in primary care relative to what could have been achieved was hard.

What is stopping the move towards better primary care? It is hard to identify any one single cause. There are many vested interests in our healthcare system, and these are organised around how things currently operate. It is not easy to change. Arguably, the position of primary care in Ireland, as in most Western healthcare systems, has become weaker relative to hospital-based and specialised care, rather than stronger.

Primary care is a strong feature of Sláintecare, the blueprint for health reform developed and published in 2017 by a special Oireachtas Committee chaired by Róisín Shortall. She had previously been a Minister of State in the Department of Health and has a fundamental grasp of primary care and its centrality to achieving health and wellbeing, and tackling social determinants of health. During that time, the Department was consumed by work on a plan to shift to a universal health insurance model along the lines of some other EU countries. That tied up many officials, took years of time and energy and ultimately did not happen. I still wonder what could have been achieved if all that time, resource, energy and brainpower had been directed towards improving primary care. The truth is, with all due respect to Sláintecare, that a seismic shift in policy and implementation is needed to really prioritise primary care and make it the centre of our healthcare system.

*   *   *

Another area I was very involved in during my years as deputy CMO was cancer care. I worked very closely on it with Tracey Conroy and Gerry Coffey and was privileged to have such dedicated colleagues. The Minister for Health, Micheál Martin, appointed me to the National Cancer Forum, a body comprising doctors, nurses, allied health professionals and patient advocacy organisations. It was chaired by Paul Redmond, a Dubliner who is now professor of surgery in Cork. One of the tasks of this forum was to review and rewrite the previous cancer strategy, updating it to what then became the Strategy for Cancer Control in Ireland, which was approved by government and published in 2006.

Evidence shows that getting the diagnosis right and developing good treatment plans is critical to good outcomes. Achieving this depends on having well-organised, sustainable multidisciplinary teams (MDTs) with sufficient throughput to maintain expertise, economies of scale and economies of scope.

Sustainable means being in a position to continuously recruit good personnel to maintain and develop the service into the long term. Before 2006, cancer services in Ireland varied between hospitals, only some of which had sustainable MDTs, and care fell short of international practice. That was clear in the comparative data at the time on cancer services and outcomes.

The precise make-up of an MDT will vary depending on the type of cancer. The key is that there is an MDT in place and that they discuss all new cancer diagnoses so that the diagnosis can be confirmed and optimised and the best course of treatment planned and final outcomes measured in the light of those plans. Delivery of treatment may happen in a more diffused way where that is appropriate; for example, chemotherapy may be administered outside of but under the direction of a cancer centre.

Our task in preparing the new strategy was, as I saw it, to design and implement a system that improved our national service relative to other countries' and that eliminated inequality in services and outcomes. The public should have the assurance of knowing they would be referred to the appropriate place by their GP or a screening service, without themselves having to understand the detail of how the cancer care system operated.

Surgery was one area of focus. We used the Hospital In-Patient Enquiry (HIPE) system, which is a national system that captures information on every admission to hospital, including the diagnosis and the types of investigations and procedures carried out. We undertook analyses to see how broadly distributed throughout our hospital system was surgical treatment for certain common cancers. In the case of breast cancer surgery, for example, we discovered there were at least 35 public hospitals carrying out surgical procedures on women with breast cancer. Of these, only five or six would have been dealing with appropriately large numbers.

Evidence has established that volume (the number of new cancers diagnosed in a centre per year) supports the development and maintenance of expertise of individuals and of the team. In breast cancer, for example, the evidence-based standard at the time was that a specialised centre should be treating at least a hundred new breast cancers a year – two per week. The policy at the time was also that a breast cancer surgeon should, ideally, manage a minimum of fifty newly diagnosed cases per year. It also specified that a surgical team should be composed of a surgical oncologist, a radiologist and a pathologist, and the three would come together as an MDT for the purpose of diagnosis and treatment planning.

Our analysis showed that these standards were not being met sufficiently. We also had good reason to believe that many women with breast cancer were not getting adjuvant (secondary or follow-up) treatment as a matter of course. In simple terms, where their treatment was happening outside the specialised centres, they were having surgery, but not necessarily chemotherapy or radiotherapy.

This analysis was a key part of the Strategy for Cancer Control in Ireland 2006. The data was clearly telling us that cancer services were scattered across too many public hospitals than should be the case. That is what had to be tackled. The cancer strategy had to focus on how services were organised and structured and how that might be impacting the quality of overall services.

* * *

Another area we put a lot of work into while I was deputy CMO was radiation oncology services, and the reorganisation of these. Tracey Conroy, Gerry Coffey and I worked closely with Professor Donal Hollywood of St James's Hospital and Trinity College. He was a committed supporter of public provision of radiation through a small number of larger centres, with radiation being fully integrated with medical and surgical oncology and all other disciplines. It was this vision that formed the basis of our policy. And that is what now exists in the new centres in St James's and Beaumont hospitals, as well as the further developments that have happened in University Hospital Galway and Cork University Hospital.

Jim Kiely led an expert panel, which included contributors from the USA, the UK and the Netherlands, on an evidence-based selection of the two sites in Dublin. It reported in 2005 and reshaped Dublin-based radiotherapy services. It was a model of impartiality and fairness. Each centre had to prepare and present a criteria-based case for the service, which led to an onsite interview by the assessment panel with each hospital. It avoided criticism of the form that was later levelled at the site selection process for the National Children's Hospital, something for which Jim deserves recognition.

Later, Emer came to use the service in St James's Hospital. She is one of many people to benefit from Donal Hollywood's vision. In fact, when Emer was diagnosed, Donal was her radiation oncologist and a key part of her MDT, which was led by Prof Paul Browne.

Donal developed cancer and sadly died in 2013 at the young age of 53. I have a particular story that really illustrates the kind of man he was. When Emer was in St James's Hospital for her stem-cell transplant, I wheeled her to the main X-ray department for a radiology procedure. We came around a corner and there was Donal, in his pyjamas and dressing gown, waiting for his own radiology procedure. As soon as he saw us, he jumped up and ran ahead of us, opening doors and making sure someone attended to Emer.

*   *   *

I travelled to Vancouver to attend an international cancer control congress hosted by the British Columbia Cancer Agency (BCCA) in late 2005. When I returned, I advised my colleagues and the Minster for Health, Mary Harney, of what was to be seen in how Canadian provinces were managing cancer control at the provincial level and how we should learn from it. A ministerial visit was arranged for February 2006 to Cancer Care Ontario (CCO) and the BCCA. That paved the way for a mentorship agreement with the BCCA to support the establishment of the National Cancer Control Programme (NCCP) to drive the implementation of the 2006 strategy we had worked on for so long. Professor Tom Keane, who was working in BCCA at the time, was appointed the first director of the NCCP.

A pivotal moment in 2007 paved the way for the implementation of Ireland's Strategy for Cancer Control. Mary Harney gathered all the leaders and stakeholders of breast cancer care in Ireland in a workshop in Farmleigh House facilitated by Olivia O'Leary. Her mission was to make it clear to everyone that they needed to be up for the challenge of reforming breast cancer management and supporting the National Cancer Control Programme and Tom Keane in implementing it. She committed her full political support, but she made that conditional on everyone being on board. Nothing like this had happened before. It was a defining moment which would change breast cancer treatment for the better.

There are now eight specialist centres for the management of breast cancer, and this has changed the way it is dealt with across the country. There is still progress to be made on other types of cancers, but much more cancer diagnosis and treatment planning is happening in specialised centres via MDTs.

The NCCP also provided the impetus for the HSE to establish other national clinical programmes. While these don't have the governance 'muscle' of the NCCP, they have made impressive improvements in the national organisation of, and outcomes related to, the treatment of stroke, coronary heart disease and epilepsy. The cancer strategy and the leadership of those involved in its development and implementation, including Mary Harney and Tom Keane, showed the way.

As far as the radiation oncology reorganisation goes, what exists now is a much better service than we had. Some of the ways in which it falls short can be attributed to the fact that the radiation oncology plan, which contained a detailed needs assessment for the future, provided an excellent business case for radiotherapy services outside the public system. The capital investment in radiation oncology is enormous. Linear accelerator machines were added to private hospitals, and made it harder to make the case for investment in further building up the larger public centres.

I would have liked to have seen more progress in the system of cancer surveillance that the 2006 strategy provided for. Monitoring, publication and open reporting of the process and outcomes of clinical care is an important promoter of change and improvement and is an integral part of a high-quality and safe service. A consistent objection is that the data quality is not good enough. But if we are to wait for perfect data before starting to measure, report and analyse, it will never happen. It is the use of data that improves the quality of data and not the other way around!

The Cancer Control Strategy of 2006 set the aim of improving our national performance relative to other countries in the EU. In November 2022, *Lancet Oncology*, a trusted and reputable journal, reported on trends in survival and outcomes for a selection of solid tumours across a number of countries. Their results show that Ireland has had above-average performance in terms of improved survival. It links this directly to that 2006 strategy, and the focus on centralisation in specialised multi-modality centres with MDT management of all cancers.

Mary Harney, as Minister for Health, made it happen and had the commitment and vision to see it through. The cancer outcomes as reported in *Lancet Oncology* are her evidence-based legacy, and independent proof that the changes were correct and necessary.

When we consider our wealth as a country, I am certain we can go further and improve more. If that is to be our national aspiration, we have to have a national cancer plan that unites clinical, academic, industry, public and private interests behind one national approach. The international context of the Cancer Moonshot initiative in the USA and Europe's Beating Cancer Plan should be seen as opportunities for Ireland to explore and exploit, not as individuals and institutions, but as a whole country.

*　*　*

Throughout those years as deputy CMO, I learned a great deal. I learned how to operate within the civil service – something that is a job in itself. I learned that not every project, no matter how worthy, will find support. And that even those projects that get adopted and resourced won't always be implemented as they should be. But, more important, I learned that change is possible. I saw that good ideas can get a fair hearing, and that, with hard work, people's lives can be affected in positive ways by the work done in the offices and at the desks of government buildings. It is a privilege, an opportunity and a responsibility to work in such a place.

CHAPTER SEVEN
Chief Medical Officer
2008

I HAD BEEN A deputy CMO for six years when the CMO, Dr Jim Kiely, announced he was leaving. There was a gap of a couple of months without a CMO, during which time we just got on with what we were doing – we had five experienced deputy CMOs at that point. The advertisement for the CMO post appeared in September 2008, and I applied. I had spent six years as deputy CMO and had had great opportunities to show what I could do. If it didn't work out, I knew I would move on with no regrets.

The advertisement made it clear that the CMO, as well as having a broad advisory role, would in future also have responsibility for patient safety and public health policy. I was attracted by that change as it meant an opportunity to take on responsibility for areas that were central to my professional training as a public health doctor.

I did the interview on a Wednesday at the very beginning of December 2008 and I found out unofficially on the following day that I had got the job. I was at home with Emer when I got a phone call to tell me the news. Emer and I were both over the moon. We had been out the night before, to a Swell Season gig in the Olympia, to take our minds off the waiting.

But now we could celebrate. We opened a nice bottle of wine we had bought that summer in Saint-Émilion on our family holiday. This was a dream come true for me. This was the highest office in public health in Ireland and I had it in my hands.

I decided I would take that Friday to finish up a few things and start the new role the following Monday. When you're an insider, as I was, it is best to move straight into the role following promotion. That is the way of things in the civil service in any case. And I think that is a good thing. I spoke to a few colleagues in the department, and other than them and my family – a really tight group of people – nobody knew. The news wasn't yet out. But before Monday arrived, an acute emergency arose out of left field.

On the Saturday morning, 6 December 2008, I was coaching kids in my GAA club, Templeogue Synge Street. I was running around with a whistle in my hand when I heard my phone. It was Minister Mary Harney. She got straight to the point. 'We're here in the Department of Agriculture. The pig flock has been contaminated with dioxins. There is poisoned pork meat for sale on the shelves. You need to come in.'

She and I had worked on a few things together by then, and I knew her pretty well. I have always held her in high regard and am happy we have stayed in touch right up to the present day. I knew what she was like as a person as well as a minister, and at first, I honestly thought it was a wind-up, a kind of initiation gag. But she kept talking, and I quickly realised it wasn't.

I already knew about a dioxin issue, related to chocolate, that had arisen in Belgium. The then ruling party and Prime Minister lost office in the general election on foot of enormous public outrage at how they handled it. The dioxin contamination in Ireland very quickly became a crisis. By teatime on

that first Saturday, I was sitting in a meeting chaired by
Taoiseach Brian Cowen. I was part of a press conference that
evening. News of the crisis went all around the world. Other
countries were naturally very quick to highlight the risks, and
thereby create opportunities for their own industries. It was
coming up to Christmas – peak pork production time – and
straightaway the pig industry went into lobbying mode.

There were two dynamics at play. One was around public
health and the protection of Irish people who had apparently
been exposed to something, although we didn't know yet
exactly what, how extensively or for how long. The second
dynamic, and of less concern to me, was the potential reputational risk of pork products, both for the domestic market and,
probably much more significantly, for the international market.

In my role, my focus is purely public health. I worked on
the assumption that the people who look after wider economic
and industry issues are good at what they do. Every government
department has its own imperatives and priorities. I was clear
on what ours was.

The first 48 hours was very intense. It taught me a great
deal about how to respond to public health emergencies,
something that was later very valuable in the context of swine
flu and, later still, Covid.

First, we needed to assemble a team of experts to advise us
on how best to deal with this. We needed to carry out a risk
assessment. My job wasn't to know about toxicology, for
example, but to assemble the people who did. All those we
called responded really generously, even though we contacted
them on Saturday night for a risk assessment meeting on Sunday
morning. The risk assessment showed that one would have to
consume large quantities of dioxin over a long period of time
to suffer significant ill effects. That was reassuring, and it helped
to inform our public messaging.

There was an immediate product recall; all pork products were pulled from the shop shelves and elsewhere. That was visually very significant, especially coming up to Christmas. That was a start. But you also have to think about people who have already bought the product but perhaps not yet consumed it. The only way to address this kind of risk is through clear public messages. You also need to consider those who have eaten the product and might, for example, be worried because they had fed it to their children. People needed somewhere to go with that worry, so we set up helplines, and briefed GPs who would be asked questions by their patients. It is also very important that politicians, as public representatives, have enough information to be able to answer questions at local level, and perhaps also use their profile to convey a consistent message of information and reassurance.

I was very focused on the messaging to the public and to GPs, and did quite an amount of it myself. After a very intense few days, it was over. People heard the messages, they saw the bare shelves, and then they saw those shelves filled again, and knew, thanks to the public health messaging, that these new products were free of dioxin contamination. We took decisive action and had clear public health messages and clear follow-up with GPs. The public was largely reassured.

I learned the value of being out there, early and visibly; telling people what we knew; telling people what we weren't certain of; telling them what we were doing and why. I saw how clear and decisive messaging could help to protect health and was also vital for building confidence for the future, including for the industry and for the Department of Agriculture.

That was a sharp introduction to my new role. There was no planned or orderly announcement of my appointment. People sent me messages saying, 'I heard you on the radio being described as the CMO . . .' They assumed the wrong title had been given. And yet, it was a good opportunity for me to get my approach to things established. One senior civil servant said to me, after an intense Sunday evening meeting at the Department of Agriculture, 'You couldn't have asked for a better opportunity to let it be known that there is a new regime.'

*   *   *

I was thrown in at the deep end of my new role so abruptly that it was several days before I moved into my new, slightly bigger, office next door to my old one. Little changed materially but there were significant changes to the structure of the position. My predecessor, Jim Kiely, had done the job on contract, initially for seven years, and then a further three years.

I was promoted to the position of CMO at 41, and offered a permanent contract until I was 65. I felt at the time I was appointed that after seven to ten years I would probably be looking for a new challenge. My belief was, and still is, that you can't be CMO for 24 years, and still be approaching it with energy and ambition at the end of that time. Inasmuch as I thought ahead, I had an idea that I might at that stage look outside the country – when you move on from the position of CMO, there aren't lots of other places to go within Ireland – and by then the children would be getting into adulthood.

Those were the sorts of feelings in my head. What actually happened was that I was in the job about three years when Emer got sick. That changed my perspective on everything. I was very glad of the permanent contract then. There was a lot of instability in our lives on the home front, so it was a blessing that we didn't also have professional instability. If I had been in a contract position, in a job that I then had to leave, it would have created a lot of upheaval, which we certainly didn't need.

*   *   *

My new role began in late 2008, at a time when the economy was in serious trouble. Those were grim times. The shutters were coming down everywhere. I learned that the role I had vacated as deputy would not be filled. That created an intense situation straight away. We were down overnight from five deputies to four, I had no resources and I knew I hadn't a hope of getting any. It was nearly 10 years before I was able to advertise for any extra person to work in the office.

I was to have executive functions in the areas of patient safety and public health as well as my advisory role. That meant those functions and their staff would move to my division from other divisions in the department. That was how I was to build up the scale of my division.

It didn't happen overnight. Discussions and negotiations with human resources absorbed most of my first two years as CMO. Frankly, it was frustrating and disheartening at times. Unions representing general civil servants were intimating that if their members were to report to me it would mean a change in their terms and conditions. It did get resolved, but only after a couple of years.

I now had a larger and more diverse team, which enabled me to take more responsibility. I believed in the importance of responsibility being passed downwards through my division by empowering and supporting people and removing fear of blame and punishment. That is what encourages people to take more responsibility. Good people respond in such an environment. I always tried to run my division on that basis. And I had really good people working with me.

CHAPTER EIGHT
Swine Flu

'THERE'S SOMETHING FUNNY GOING on in Mexico ...' Dr Derval Igoe said when I answered her call late on Friday afternoon, 24 April 2009. I was still less than six months in the role. Derval, a senior and well-respected public health doctor in the HPSC, said there had been reports of cases of a new strain of influenza that appeared to be passing from pigs to humans. An alert had been received through the WHO (World Health Organization) early warning system for sharing such information.

The USA was already expressing alarm. In June 2009, about six weeks after the initial report, the WHO officially declared a pandemic of influenza A (H1N1), which came to be commonly known as swine flu. 'Pandemic' means that a disease has reached epidemic level in at least two of the six regions of the WHO. That declaration has important implications within the WHO for the release of resources and the organisation of work priorities.

My first concern was to get our governance arrangements and communication strategy right. At the time, pandemic planning had been undertaken in line with the national strategy on emergency planning in accordance with WHO guidelines. One key structure that was in existence as a result was the National Pandemic Influenza Expert Group (PIEG), established in 2003 and chaired by Professor Bill Hall, Dr Cillian de Gascun's predecessor. Advice provided by this group was central to the development of the National Pandemic Influenza Plan, which was the plan that in turn informed many of our actions.

A National Public Health Emergency Team (NPHET) was established. In the initial weeks, it had a daily meeting followed by a press conference. I now realise that daily meetings were probably excessive, but initially, in the first stages of the pandemic, we wanted to get control quickly, as far as anyone could, of the assessment process – what we assessed this threat to be and what measures were needed – and the clear communication of information.

The first case of swine flu in Ireland was identified on 5 May 2009. By 1 July, fifty cases had been confirmed. There was genuine public fear, influenced early on by reports of deaths that were related to swine flu. There were thankfully few of these, but they were nonetheless concerning.

We were open in press briefings and media interviews with the information we had, and deliberately vague about specific details of cases. The basic outline was all we gave: for example male or female, adult or child. The media were irritated that we wouldn't tell them more. But we saw it as our duty to provide enough detail to enable the public to take actions that were appropriate, but not so much that confidentiality would be compromised. After a time, the media stopped asking about individual cases.

With swine flu, media interest never really extended beyond health correspondents. There was also limited interest in the wider political system. Mary Harney, however, as Minister for Health, and Tánaiste at the time, was interested. She wasn't a micro-manager and was inclined to trust in our ability to do our jobs. And in broad terms we managed our response to that first wave of swine flu reasonably well. It wasn't perfect. We did what was required. I learned a great deal from that experience. We responded to the information we had at each moment. Vaccines became available and were delivered. In the winter of 2009, there was a second potentially more severe wave, a pattern we would have anticipated. Over the following years, waves of swine flu gave way to the virus becoming one of the seasonal influenza strains and against which annual influenza vaccines provide cover.

It became clear that older sections of the population were less susceptible. Immunity most likely resulted from previous influenza infections and therefore meant that older adults were relatively more protected. Children, however, were particularly vulnerable. There were over one thousand confirmed swine flu admissions to hospital. Almost ten per cent of these were to intensive care units (ICUs). The highest admission rates were in the under-fives. We came very close to exceeding ICU capacity in Dublin paediatric hospitals. Very ill children experienced cancelled or delayed procedures, including cardiac surgery. It is easy to forget that.

From late April 2009, Ireland operated a containment phase, which involved early detection, isolation and treatment of suspected cases as well as contact tracing to limit the spread of the virus. In addition, extra supplies and equipment were purchased during this period, including vaccines and anti-viral medications, as well as essential equipment such as ventilators and dialysis units.

In mid-July 2009, the strategy moved from containment to a mitigation phase when it was no longer feasible to contact trace all cases. The aim of the mitigation strategy was to limit the impact of the virus on the population through public information, use of anti-virals and vaccination. Two vaccines were authorised for use. The HSE set up mass vaccination clinics. In the early months, we saw a high uptake of vaccines compared to other countries. When the public began to understand that swine flu was not as serious as had initially appeared, vaccination uptake dropped very significantly.

*   *   *

Early on, it became clear that Ireland would not get access to new swine flu vaccines that were being developed without an advance purchase agreement (APA) in place. We had to pay to queue. We also had to accept an indemnification clause as part of an APA, which is a relatively standard component of contracts between vaccine manufacturers and government purchasers.

I do have questions about the ethics of such arrangements, but the truth is that this is how the market works. It is also true that not being in that priority queue could have had very serious consequences. The same system applied with Covid-19 vaccines. Ireland was part of a common EU procurement of vaccines, which meant that Ireland had access to Covid vaccines at the same time as the rest of Europe.

The initial consignment of swine flu pandemic vaccine (36,000 doses) arrived in the first week of September 2009. The vaccination strategy prioritised high-risk groups and healthcare workers, followed by schoolchildren. The vaccination of over-65-year-olds began in early December 2009 and thereafter the vaccine was offered to the rest of the population from the beginning of February 2010. The public pandemic vaccination campaign ended on 31 March 2010. The vaccine continued to be made available free of charge to the various 'at risk' groups until September 2010.

A few months into the vaccination roll-out, case reports began to emerge around the world of a larger than usual number of children diagnosed with narcolepsy, a chronic neurological disorder that affects control of sleep. It was picked up through pharmacovigilance, which is the detection, assessment, monitoring and prevention of adverse effects relating to pharmaceutical products. It includes analysis of reports of side effects that may be related to a new medicine, after the medicine or vaccine is licensed, to determine whether they are in line with the expected profile of side effects.

Clinical trials for vaccines are designed to detect common side effects and to ensure that the vaccine produces the required immune response in those vaccinated. A side effect or a complication of a medication or vaccine that has been through all appropriate safety trials and authorisation processes can sometimes be found to have a delayed effect or an effect at such a low level of incidence that it would not have been detectable in the initial clinical trials. Use of a vaccine which has the potential to save lives and prevent serious illness cannot be delayed by virtue of a very small possibility of a rare event that may also take years to emerge.

As cases of narcolepsy began to appear and there were reports of a possible link, our focus was understanding any medical needs that might arise. A group was set up in May 2011, chaired by Dr Joe Devlin, HSE Clinical Director Quality and Patient Safety. This group planned and co-ordinated the service response from the HSE and included patient liaison and other supports. It worked closely with SOUND, a group of parents of children with narcolepsy or cataplexy (sudden muscular weakness), which often goes with narcolepsy.

The HSE put in place a system of care to have these children assessed and treated, without the requirement for them to establish how their particular illness might have arisen. If a case of childhood narcolepsy was suspected, the child would be referred through this pathway to HSE services, and fast-tracked to ensure access to treatment as speedily as possible.

* * *

Looking back at the response to the swine flu vaccination programme I would say that on the basis of the information we had at each point in time, as a country we responded well and proportionately. Over 1.1 million pandemic vaccinations were recorded, giving a 25 per cent uptake for the total population. The evidence of the impact of the second and successive waves of swine flu shows that our vaccination levels protected public health in Ireland well as compared to other countries.

It was not all perfect and I'm sure we didn't get everything right. Decisions can only be made with the information that is available at the time. This information is often incomplete and far from perfect. Protecting public health during an emergency such as a pandemic means making the best decisions possible in spite of limited information. Certainly there were mistakes that I learned from and rectified in the Covid pandemic.

One was the frequency with which we ran the NPHET meetings during the swine flu pandemic. For a long period, they took place daily. That was too often. Separating out the issues that needed daily attention from those that needed less frequent attention and ensuring that there were integrated processes for each would have made it easier to manage. The same doesn't apply, however, to press communication. Daily communication, when the pandemic was at its most intense, was, I think, something we did get right and was something I learned and carried with me to the Covid response.

Another mistake we made was inadequately documenting what we were doing. This became clearer to me over time, particularly when legal discovery orders relating to narcolepsy had to be carried out. The system of minutes, agendas, documentation and recording of clear decisions and advice was too weak. At the time, I didn't realise the central importance of that, and that was definitely a mistake.

This is something I was particularly careful not to repeat during the Covid pandemic. In the initial weeks of Covid, getting minutes turned around was slower than I wanted it to be. We quickly mobilised resources to make it a priority. As well as trying to respond to a rapidly unfolding crisis, we were trying to assemble the team, get our response off the ground, and document everything that we did and discussed. As a result, there is a detailed public record online of who was at every NPHET meeting, what was discussed, what was agreed, what recommendations and advice were to be provided, and a detailed letter of advice was sent to the minister after each meeting.

* * *

A final word about swine flu. My children became the first two children in St Pius X Boys' and Girls' national schools in Terenure to be confirmed with swine flu; this was during the first week of September 2009. I have no idea where they picked it up. They were off school for about a week. Ronan was seven and Clodagh was eight at the time.

Emer was also infected and was sick enough to go to the emergency department, where a swab confirmed the diagnosis and showed she had a severe chest infection. She was almost fully confined to bed. Her mother, Ita, called to the house every day for three or four days and left shopping at the door. I was working 16-hour days and somehow managed to avoid the illness completely. Clodagh was moderately ill but Ronan had almost no symptoms. He must have thought all his Sundays had come at once. He was a PlayStation whizz at the end of it!

CHAPTER NINE
Emer's Diagnosis
2012

EMER WAS DIAGNOSED WITH multiple myeloma in September 2012. The months leading up to the diagnosis are some of the hardest parts of those very difficult years to revisit. The length of time her diagnosis took, the false reassurance we received along the way, and the stage her cancer had reached by the time she was finally diagnosed, all caused very great distress to her, to the children and to me.

Emer found it very hard to accept the early handling of her symptoms. The story of her delayed diagnosis is one she wanted to be told. Illness happens and tragedies occur all too often, and as I have already mentioned, medical errors are also common. These can affect anyone. There may be comfort for others to learn that these things happen indiscriminately. Having medical knowledge, even a certain position within the medical community, does not insure you against error or harm. Certainly, I believe that in Emer's case it did not.

My first recollection of Emer experiencing severe pain was Easter 2012. We were in Malaga airport. We had just arrived, with Clodagh and Ronan, who were nine and eleven, for a short holiday at the Sunset Beach Club in Benalmádena, a favourite destination for many Irish families. It is a place we have been to many times and has happy memories for us as a family. When lifting a bag, Emer hurt a rib and we believed it was a muscular injury. She was in pain for much of the holiday. But with analgesia and rest, that pain subsided in the following week or two.

In early June 2012, Emer had a further similar episode of rib cage pain, which was tender to the touch. I referred her by letter to a hospital emergency department (ED). Emer was seen by a senior doctor who didn't carry out any investigations and reassured her, based on a clinical examination (i.e. a clinical assessment without the use of diagnostic tests), that her condition was likely to be a benign self-limiting one.

We now know it wasn't benign. In retrospect we know her rib pain was probably caused by a rib fracture, in turn caused by myeloma, but this wasn't diagnosed until much later. Emer came home after that ED visit reassured that this was nothing serious, an intercostal muscle strain perhaps; something that needed rest and simple analgesia and no more. And indeed, the pain settled down because the rib injury healed.

In late August 2012, she had a further episode, which caused me to refer her to the same ED. This time she had severe pain in her spine and shoulder blade. She was also complaining of tingling in her fingers which was relieved by moving her arms. I made sure to reference several episodes of rib pain over the preceding months in my referral letter. She was seen by a different consultant. She was again told, without the benefit of any tests and with only a clinical assessment, that there was nothing to worry about. This time, she was less reassured. I think she had a sense that something more was wrong. But she tried to carry on with life, work, and the children.

It is my view that Emer should have had some basic tests carried out on each occasion she went to the ED. I simply do not understand the decision to carry out no investigation when

Emer re-presented with persistent and more extensive symptoms in late August. Myeloma is often picked up by chance, and before a patient develops symptoms, when an abnormality is found on a routine blood test or X-ray carried out for other purposes. There is no way of knowing with certainty if simple tests such as these would have shown some abnormality. I think it is reasonable, however, to suggest that they would, if not in early June, then very probably in late August. And that would have made an enormous difference to Emer.

I have no doubt that the resultant delay in diagnosis resulted in her being much sicker, risking her life and experiencing much more pain than if she'd been diagnosed after that first, or even second, ED visit. Looking back, it is hard for me to think about the faith I placed in the reassurance that there was nothing serious behind her symptoms.

Myeloma is not a curable disease. I am not saying that an earlier diagnosis would have saved Emer's life. Alas, that couldn't have been the case. But she had a very difficult course with her disease, particularly in its initial presentation and the extent of the bone disease that she had. She suffered greatly with horrific bone pain for eight years. It was difficult for her to function without pain. She certainly suffered far more than she would have with an earlier diagnosis.

Emer was very upset about this. It became something that preoccupied her and caused her great unhappiness. This was mostly because of how much it affected her time with the children, and her ability to do things with them and be there for them as she wanted to be and when they needed her to be. Later, she wrote a detailed letter of complaint to the hospital, describing her experiences, and the impact of them on her life. She was extremely open and honest about the cost to her. I think expressing her views in writing was helpful to her.

In return, however, we received a response that was disappointing. It suggested that matters of clinical judgement by doctors were not matters for the hospital – implying but not stating that such complaints were perhaps for some other unidentified authority such as the Medical Council or perhaps a court. Emer had no desire to go down either of these difficult avenues. She simply wanted the hospital to acknowledge and learn from her experience. But the hospital had no plan to take the matter further, apparently. It proposed no examination of or changes to procedures, for example, that might be applied to repeat attendances. It did not explain why it saw a matter of clinical judgement as falling outside its area of responsibility.

Professional performance of clinical duties, including judgements by doctors, should be an accepted part of the health service responsibility to every patient. Each episode of harm to a patient must be seen as an opportunity to learn and improve. A mistake by a doctor does not imply incompetence and, for Emer, professional competence was not in question in this case. Most questions about performance of clinical duties or judgement do not raise questions of competence on the part of a doctor. But that does not imply that hospitals and health service providers can simply, in effect, leave it to the individual, who may already be harmed, vulnerable and upset.

The Irish Medical Council undertook, some years ago, a very worthwhile but concerning analysis of complaints it had received. It showed that a very small proportion of individual patient complaints about professional performance led to significant sanction. It also showed that it is unusual for a health service organisation or hospital to become a complainant in a matter of poor performance in relation to one of its own doctors. The net effect of all this is that many patients who suffer harm are left in limbo. Unless their case is extremely serious, the Medical Council is unlikely to take action and the health service provider takes no action because clinical judgement is declared not to be a matter for them.

Court judgments in well-known legal cases in Ireland show that complaints of poor performance to the Medical Council cannot easily be substantiated by individual cases. This is an impossibly high standard for an individual patient with a complaint. Poor performance as a standard in the context of medical practice therefore effectively only applies to a series of cases that show patterns of consistent poor performance. Only a hospital or health service provider is in a position to create such evidential basis for a complaint to the Medical Council relating to poor professional performance – yet here was a hospital stating that the matters of clinical judgement in Emer's case were not matters within its own responsibility to Emer.

Health service providers and hospitals ought to know better. Many health service providers and hospitals do not appear to see it as their duty or responsibility to routinely monitor professional performance among doctors. There is no system in place to ensure that doctors who repeatedly fall below professional standards are systematically identified and appropriate remediation measures put in place. This established culture and practice, which was reflected in the letter to Emer, makes no sense in a modern understanding of patient safety.

I am aware that the HSE, to its credit, has established escalation procedures relating to clinical complaints. Legislation and updated patient safety practices and processes are, in my view, required to better support open disclosure, monitoring and assurance of quality, incident investigation and learning from possible errors and harms to patients. That might not have prevented what happened to Emer, but it would have yielded a more satisfactory response to her complaint.

I still find this very hard to think about. But I think it is important to write about this, because there will be other people who have had similar experiences. And perhaps the knowledge that this can – and does – happen to anyone may be of some comfort.

*　　*　　*

In early September 2012, I was on a two-day work trip to Malta, to the Standing Committee Meeting of the WHO Euro Region. At that stage, I was travelling to international meetings as part of my job. It was to be the last international meeting I attended as CMO. I never travelled again for work purposes while Emer was still alive.

I remember talking to Emer about whether I should go or not, because of her recent pain, but she had been feeling better over the preceding days and was adamant that I should. I flew over on a Sunday and on the Monday morning Ronan rang me to say, 'Mam is not able to come down the stairs.' This was a new development. He brought the phone to Emer and we spoke. I decided to come home immediately. I rang Pauline, my secretary, and asked her to get me the next flight home. I then phoned a GP friend of mine, Barry Quinn, and said 'Emer is in trouble, would you see her?' From that day onwards, he cared for Emer for the rest of her life. She couldn't have wished for a better GP. Emer loved him and had great faith in him.

I was concerned, obviously, but I wasn't thinking about cancer. I was thinking of arthritic conditions, something like rheumatoid arthritis perhaps, which would be serious enough; but perhaps I was not prepared to let myself think about the worst possible case. While waiting in Malta airport for a flight to Düsseldorf, from where I would connect to Dublin, I spoke to Barry. He had just seen Emer. He had taken bloods and sent them to the laboratory and said he would be in touch as soon as he got the results back. He was worried. That rattled me. But I spoke to Emer and told her I was on my way, and would be home by evening. She was feeling a bit better by then, having seen Barry.

By the time Barry rang back, I was on the plane in Düsseldorf, ready to take off for Dublin. I took the call. I had left my phone on until the last minute for this very reason. I'll never forget that conversation. He had the blood results. Emer's haemoglobin was 10 and her erythrocyte sedimentation rate (ESR) – a crude measure of inflammation – was 100. I knew immediately that we were in trouble. These are two markers of chronic illness and both were very concerning. The results meant that Emer was anaemic, and she had some very significant inflammatory process happening. There had to be something very sinister and organic going on.

I asked Barry to say nothing to Emer, to let me tell her. I hung up, and immediately rang Martha. Thank goodness she answered quickly because the air steward was now practically standing over me, requesting that I turn my phone off. I tearfully blurted out the basic facts to Martha, and she immediately said, 'Don't worry, I'm on it. It will be sorted.'

By the time I landed in Dublin that Monday evening, there was a bed booked in St Vincent's Private Hospital for the following morning under the care of Dr Hugh Mulcahy, Martha's husband. The key was to get Emer in quickly and start the process of investigation, even though Hugh knew that his field – gastroenterology – probably wasn't the expertise Emer might finally require.

Then I had to tell Emer. It was late when I arrived home from the airport and the children were asleep. I went into the playroom, where Emer was watching television. I can still see her expression as I came through the door. Fear and forced smiles on both our faces. I told her about the blood results. Emer knew their significance. Of course she did.

Emer was first admitted to hospital on Tuesday 11 September 2012. We still hoped it might be a disorder like rheumatoid arthritis or lupus, for example. Either of those would be bad, but not in comparison with other possibilities. But quickly it became clear that we weren't going to be so lucky.

I had to collect a hard copy of the blood results from Barry on the Wednesday morning, to bring them to St Vincent's. He said he thought myeloma was a strong possibility. That was the first mention of it and it really shook me. Barry told me about another young patient he had seen present with it, years previously, and the impression it had made on him. Emer reminded him of this.

I cried all the way to St Vincent's.

By that evening we knew Emer had cancer. I can still remember hearing Hugh Mulcahy walk down the corridor towards Emer's room; the sound of his shoes on the hard floor, the heaviness of his pace. He had the terrible task of coming to us with the results of a CT scan. I can still hear him delivering the news: 'I'm sorry, the scan is not normal.'

Among the possibilities, he said, were a widely disseminated cancer like melanoma or perhaps multiple myeloma. Emer needed a bone biopsy to determine precisely what kind of cancer this was. The biopsy was carried out and results weren't due to be available until after the weekend, but the pathologist very kindly came in on Saturday morning to examine the biopsy and give us the definitive diagnosis.

We were trying to keep life as normal as possible for Clodagh and Ronan, who were then aged eleven and nine, through that awful week. Ronan was playing and I was coaching at a club match in Ballyboden St Enda's when the call came to confirm myeloma. Such is the surreal nature of serious illness, I also remember thinking in relief, 'Okay, it's myeloma.' If it had been a widely disseminated cancer Emer probably would have had a very limited life span. With myeloma, if we could treat it successfully, Emer might have a few years. This felt like a fighting chance.

I could hear and feel the relief and resolve in Emer. We had certainty back in our lives. She now knew what she was dealing with and what her priorities were. Emer had some things going for her. She was young, otherwise healthy, and had many resources available to deal with the treatment and the disease itself. I remember that it was she who comforted me, and not the other way around. It was Emer who said, 'We'll be okay,' Emer who vowed that she would fight for every extra day, to be with the children.

CHAPTER TEN
Everything Changes
2012

WHAT WE WENT THROUGH as a family in the years after Emer's diagnosis, during her illness and up to her death, are things that I can talk about. But I am very aware that beyond that is the separate story of what Emer herself went through. There are hardships that I only know of through what she told me and through what she wrote to me and to the children: reflections, guidance, thoughts for after she was gone.

I try to bring these things with me while I write this book, knowing well that I can only ever be partly successful. I can't fully speak, or write, for Emer, and I think it is important that I acknowledge that. But I can try to share something of her experiences. This is something she wanted me to do.

Doing that is difficult. But it isn't anything like as difficult as losing her. We've been through the worst of it. Going back over it now for this book is bearable, in comparison.

* * *

I have only partial memories of that Wednesday evening in St Vincent's when Hugh confirmed it was cancer and suggested myeloma as the most likely form. I remember Emer's strength.

She didn't go to pieces. She was the one holding my hand, the one saying we'd be okay.

I know from my training and clinical days, and have often heard it said by patients, that when they're given bad news, they take in only a tiny bit of the information. That day, I experienced the truth of that.

Multiple myeloma causes multiple deposits or lesions, called myelomas, mostly in bone marrow, which means that it usually appears in marrow-containing bones. These deposits of myeloma, depending on where they are, cause local effects. It is not a common cancer, and it generally affects older people. It accounts for about 1 per cent of all cancers, and only 5 per cent of cancers in the under-50s. Normally, the age of onset would be in the over-70s. Three decades older than Emer, who was only 45.

When we had both absorbed the news, the next step was to tell the children. By then, Clodagh and Ronan knew that a cancer diagnosis was a possibility. We had kept them informed at each step along the way and kept the conversation with them as open as we could. As a parent you would do anything to avoid hurt or harm to your children. But Emer and I believed that uncertainty would be worse for them. Emer's diagnosis was something we couldn't protect Clodagh and Ronan from. They were both so young – Ronan was nine, Clodagh eleven – but they were old enough to know the word 'cancer' and to have some understanding of what it meant.

I read up about talking to children about cancer. I found very useful resources on the internet, and was in contact with the Irish Cancer Society. They have an excellent publication called *Talking to Children about Cancer*, which emphasises the importance of keeping children informed and involved, and being aware that they have fears they don't always articulate. Children understand very quickly when something unusual is going on, or when there is something you're not telling them. And they fill those empty spaces with conjecture. Their fears can be responded to, as long as you know that there's something you need to respond to.

On Thursday 13 September, the day after we learned Emer had cancer, I picked up Clodagh and Ronan from school and we went directly to St Vincent's, to Emer, so we could break the news to them early and together. Emer and I had talked about this and planned it together over the course of the previous evening. We told them and they cried. I remember them climbing on to Emer's bed and hugging her, but it is hard to recall the details of the conversation. Emer was magnificent. Listening to Clodagh and Ronan, watching their reactions. Not avoiding anything and answering every question they asked. We did our best to anticipate the things that might have been on their minds and we raised them. Throughout it all she maintained her composure. There was hardly a more difficult day in all the time she was unwell.

They knew about Emer's back pain, so that was how we talked about it. They knew Emer was in hospital to find out what was causing the pain, and now we were revealing that it was cancer. Ronan asked, 'Is back cancer serious?' That is how he was able to frame it.

In the evening, I brought them home. Clodagh later told me that she has a vivid recollection of that day, and particularly the drive home. She remembers looking out of the car window at the houses, and thinking about all the people living in them whose lives were simply carrying on as normal while hers had changed so much and so suddenly; how oblivious all those people were to the tragedy that had befallen our family.

And, because she is Clodagh, and because life somehow carries on, even when the most terrible things happen, she also remembers that we stopped for a treat in Wilde & Greene on our way, and she got a cupcake and a can of something fizzy.

* * *

Over those days and early weeks, I had a system whereby I would update one person in each family – Emer's and mine – so that they could update the other members of the family. That really helped me. Keeping people up to date is time-consuming and takes energy. Yet it is so important for everyone to know what is happening. I talked to Emer's sister Orla, to whom I have always been close, and did the same in my family, although it varied as to which of my five sisters I spoke to. Often it was circumstances or a phone not answered that dictated which one.

I also told Emer's parents, Frank and Ita, and family everything we knew as we knew it. Her parents were in their early 80s but still active and capable. Through all those early days, when I was in hospital, they helped with babysitting. That was the help I needed most. Without them I wouldn't have been able to get through it at all.

I had already phoned the secretary general, in the earlier part of that week, to explain the situation. I realised he had told James Reilly, then Minister for Health, when I got a call from him to say he was very sorry to hear what we were going through, and to take all the time I needed. As a doctor, he knew what life would have been like for us. That was a decent thing for him to do, and it meant that I knew that work need not be an immediate concern. All my energy was for Emer and the children.

I know what a privilege that is. If you're running your own business, for example, that simply isn't an option. With the support I had at home, I could find a good balance. I only missed one management meeting over the course of those three weeks while Emer was in hospital. I dropped into the office around visits to the hospital, and I used phone and email when I needed to. I was lucky that I had a good team of people around me and so I delegated far more than I might otherwise have been able to.

I worked out a routine. I would go into Emer in the morning, then on into work. I would call back to her later in the afternoon or evening, and I would try to collect the kids from school at least some of the days. On the days when I couldn't, Emer's parents would take over.

*   *   *

Once we realised the diagnosis was likely to be myeloma, I wanted to have Emer transferred to St James's Hospital. I spoke with Paul Browne, a senior haematologist in St James's who specialises in myeloma, and asked if he would take over her care. He agreed immediately. I knew that a bone marrow transplant was a possibility, and St James's was where she would be best placed for that. Also, it was a lot closer to where we live – 15 minutes as opposed to 30 or 40. Emer had long, extended stays in hospital over the next years and there were many days when I would drive in and back two or three times, trying to juggle home, work and being with her.

I think it is important to say that Emer didn't get prioritised ahead of anyone else. She was acutely unwell and needed urgent care. She was already in hospital, already in the system, and was always going to get that urgent care. Throughout the eight years of her illness, Emer received the same standard of care in St James's Hospital that anyone presenting with her disease would get. I believe it is important to highlight that, and I know she would want me to.

It is only in retrospect that I understand how sick she was at the time of her diagnosis and how worried Prof Browne was about her. The focus in that first week was on completing the examinations and tests to provide a complete diagnosis, and then focusing on symptom control. That meant pain control using morphine-related drugs, and radiotherapy to deal with the specific local effects of the different lesions.

The treatment causes a lot of inflammation and release of toxins called cytokines. More inflammation in the short term can paradoxically lead to more pain. So Emer's pain, which was already searing and constant, actually increased for a time. She couldn't sleep, could hardly walk, and was in truly unbearable pain.

St James's was the right place for the management of her disease; the focus was disease control treatments such as chemotherapy and radiotherapy. The primary focus is not pain and the control of symptoms per se. That is not to say the medical staff are callous or uncaring. Rather, it means that there are other doctors, palliative care doctors, who are more expert in pain and symptom management and who have that as their primary focus.

Emer raised the question of engaging the palliative care team with Prof Browne at that initial stage. She had a deep understanding of the role and value of palliative care and the importance of having it available early in the course of a cancer diagnosis. Prof Browne arranged for Emer to be attended by Dr Norma O'Leary, a truly amazing consultant. She became Emer's palliative care doctor throughout Emer's illness right up to when she died.

The role of palliative care is in control of symptoms such as pain. Clearly that becomes more important as an illness progresses, but the earlier it commences the better. Many people equate palliative care with end-of-life care and want to avoid it for that reason. Sadly, that means they sometimes deny themselves the benefit that comes from better control of symptoms and an enhanced quality of life.

*   *   *

Quite early in the process, the question of what my role was to be came up – was it to be Emer's husband, her doctor or both? I talked this out with my great friend Colin Doherty. I realised that it wouldn't be right for me to try to be Emer's 'doctor'. She was surrounded by excellent doctors in whom she had great faith. But I was the only person who could be her husband. So that's what I needed to be.

As Emer's husband my role was simply to be with her. To help her remember, interpret and understand what she was told, to support her in every way I could. It was important for us to understand what we were being told, but to also have faith – informed faith – in the people looking after her. Trust and faith in her medical team would be essential to ensuring as good an outcome as possible for Emer. I therefore saw my expertise and experience as enabling me to identify who and what to place our trust in. I felt confident that we had put our faith in the right people and the right service. Having done that, we would let them do their jobs and not second-guess them. I was a full-time husband, dad and CMO. That was enough for me to focus on.

*   *   *

I had chosen to cut out international travel and to minimise extracurricular work activities such as conferences, meetings and formal invitations. I had no choice since I had to protect my time for Emer, the family and my job. One way I could stay close to Emer and our children was as a volunteer. Both

Emer and I strongly believed in the value of volunteering and I hope we managed to pass that value to our children.

No community can operate without voluntary effort. I took on voluntary roles in the Terenure community and I was supported in this by Emer. I spent four wonderful years from 2010 on the board of management of Ronan's primary school, St Pius X Boys' National School, Terenure. The board was chaired by my good friend Ronan McMahon. It was a great school with a wonderfully charismatic and dedicated principal, Dermot Lynch – a West Cork man to his fingertips.

I also spent three years on the board of management of Clodagh's secondary school, Our Lady's School in Terenure. That was where Emer and her sisters attended and where Emer first met Martha. Emer was really very excited at the idea of me being on the board of her former school. The chair was a lovely Galway man, Kevin O'Brien, who had been principal of Templeogue College but was by now retired. The principal was Pauline Meaney, the epitome of professionalism and competence. Emer used to joke that if I wasn't on the board of the school and we were depending on Clodagh to know what was happening there, everything would be simply 'fine'. Anyone who has or had teenage children will understand that one!

The other part of my volunteering life was in my local GAA club, Templeogue Synge Street, where I coached Gaelic football for over ten years. This club was created from the amalgamation of a local juvenile club, Templeogue, and Synge Street past pupils' club. There is a family connection here in that Frank, Emer's beloved dad, who died in February 2023, was a past pupil.

My coaching career began one Saturday morning during Ronan's first few weeks at the club nursery for five-year-olds in Bushy Park, Terenure. The club's games promotion officer (a role funded by the Dublin County Board to support clubs and local schools) was a Wexford man, Ciaran Deely – Wexford football captain at the time and one of the nicest people you could meet. Ciaran asked me to help him carry a couple of bags while I was standing by. Before I knew what was happening, I had a whistle in my mouth! Looking back on it, Ciaran was a great leader and he knew well what he was doing.

I went on to coach that 2002 boys' team – which included my son Ronan, now in the senior squad – with my good friend Ronan Devitt. I kept going with the team until they were under-15s, which was about the time Emer was first admitted to the hospice. Ronan Devitt was one of a great team of mentors who led that group to win both their under-16 league and the Dublin Minor B Division championship.

Volunteering provides an opportunity to connect with others who share similar interests and values, and it has enriched my life. I've seen first-hand the benefits that volunteering can bring not only to communities but also to the individual who volunteers. There is good evidence that volunteering is very good for physical and mental health while also making a positive impact on others and on the community. For many people, it can help reduce feelings of loneliness and isolation. Volunteering has been linked to reduced symptoms of depression and anxiety, as well as improved overall mental wellbeing. It can also help reduce stress levels, as it provides a sense of control and a distraction from personal issues. This was very true in my case. To a group of young boys in a football team, you are the coach. You get no credit for anything else. They take you as they find you. And I found that refreshing.

* * *

One of the issues that arose early on after Emer's diagnosis was that her T2 vertebra, at the base of the neck, was already practically obliterated by the disease. That gave rise to a question about the stability of her neck. This time, she was referred to the Mater (while still an in-patient in St James's Hospital), and seen by Mr Ashley Poynton, an expert in the spine. He made an assessment that there was sufficient stability not to endanger her spinal cord. It was a relief to avoid surgery that time.

The possibility of surgery arose several more times over the years in relation to lesions in various parts of Emer's body. The aim of any such surgery would have been to provide stability to damaged bones. Outcomes from orthopaedic surgery in myeloma, even in the best hands, are never certain. Such surgery is far from straightforward and neither is the recovery. Emer faced the question a number of times but managed to avoid ever having orthopaedic surgery, which was great.

*   *   *

I remember a woman who, seeing me outside the school gates waiting to collect Clodagh on one of those early terrible days, called over, 'Cheer up, it might never happen!' Of course, she had no idea what had already happened. In the following weeks, I found myself running into people in the locality much more than usual because I was prioritising picking the children up from school, which was a new thing for me. And most were wonderful, sympathetic, understanding and supportive – even those we didn't know well. A woman who had recently moved in nearby called one day. She almost couldn't speak, she was so upset for us; she just handed me a pot of spaghetti Bolognese. You feel every ounce of the love and support of people like that. After a while, we had so much food in the freezer from friends, family and neighbours, I had to gently ask them to stop. But I will never forget the kindness of all those people.

One of the things I like to do is cook. I'm not saying I'm great, but I do cook, and I enjoy it. It gives me a sense of achieving something tangible, and keeps me connected to the kids. It keeps the communication going, even if it's just 'What's for dinner, Dad?'

Most people were wonderful in just that way. They step up. But it is also true that some step back. There were a couple of people who never really spoke to Emer again after she became unwell. They avoided her. I assume they didn't know what to say. Maybe Emer's illness had echoes of difficult times in their own lives. And it is also important to acknowledge that not everyone feels equipped for what they might regard as a difficult conversation. I'm sure there were reasons, but Emer was hurt by that.

And then there were those who were driven by sheer idle curiosity. Emer described answering the door to a woman one evening who had called 'with a cheesecake and a question', as Emer put it. She asked, straight out on the doorstep, 'What is your prognosis?' A question some of Emer's closest friends had the tact not to ask. That really upset Emer, but I know she didn't let that woman see it.

Martha had been diagnosed with breast cancer about a year before Emer's diagnosis. She was a wonderful guide in navigating some of the unexpected fall-out. I remember her telling Emer, 'The only good thing about all this is you don't have to talk to anyone you don't want to. Assume they'll understand. And if they don't, too bad.'

*   *   *

Once Emer came home from St James's Hospital after that initial three-week stay, she had two or three further admissions within a few months. These were shorter, and they were sudden, due to temperatures and infections. She was very vulnerable to infection as a result of very low white blood cell counts due to her treatment, so this could happen without much warning.

I always associate the television series *Love/Hate* with this time. Emer and I used to watch that together on Sunday evenings, and there were two almost identical times – each during an episode of *Love/Hate* – when she ended up feeling very unwell and had to be urgently admitted to St James's. I can remember the sick feeling of fear in the pit of my stomach as I drove her, a feeling that would become all too familiar.

Those were difficult times. The children would have gone to bed, so they would wake in the morning and find Emer was gone. That was very upsetting for them. And it was also upsetting for Emer, because she knew they would go to bed every night worrying if she would be there when they woke up. We had to really address that with them. Again, in this situation, we told them what we could. We explained white cells and their role in infection. We explained the risk of infection and the importance of speed when it is suspected. We reassured them when her white cell count was good. We didn't try to hide anything. It was as much reassurance as we could give. We tried to let them know that anything they felt or feared should be articulated. We told them that there were no stupid questions and that sometimes we would have simple answers to things they wondered about and sometimes we wouldn't, but we would always do our best to tell them what we could.

* * *

The median survival for the stage of Emer's myeloma when she was diagnosed was about three years. I remember thinking, based on everything I heard and read, if she got three to five years, we'd be doing well. She ended up having eight and a half years.

The programme of initial treatment, called induction treatment, that Emer received was aimed at getting control of the disease, and hopefully getting her well enough for a stem cell transplant. A stem cell transplant uses either your own stem cells or donated ones. In Emer's case, it was deemed preferable to use her own stem cells, although it may be different for other patients and other types of cancer. Stem cells are harvested from blood, then a drug called melphalan is given that destroys the bone marrow. The stem cells are reintroduced, to grow new and healthier bone marrow, and the hope is that for a period of time – a long period of time – this will induce remission.

*   *   *

One of the constant themes for Emer was her longing to see Clodagh and Ronan grow up, and hopefully to see them through secondary school at least. Her world shrank to being just about family and the kids. I saw my role as being to support and enable that as much as I possibly could. One of the fears she frequently expressed was that she would never get to see what Ronan looked like as a man or Clodagh as a woman. But she did get to see it. Ronan was 18 when she died, and Clodagh was 20.

That was the business of our house and family for all those years. It meant shutting down a lot of other things. We had a limited social life anyway by then – our lives were already focused very much on the kids. But life continued, that's the point. It did because it had to.

I can recall summer holidays in France or Italy over many years before Emer's illness. My mind goes easily to the four of us together in a car driving on a European motorway. I would feel so safe and happy in those moments, like nothing could touch us or get in the way of our happiness. When we were together like that, life felt wonderful.

Something did get in the way. Cancer was like an unwanted guest that moved in and wouldn't leave. We needed to figure out how to live with it. We weren't going to completely change our lives. We couldn't. The children had to go to school, lunches had to be made, clothes had to be washed and ironed, shopping done . . . And that domestic routine becomes intensely precious. That is how we felt about it, anyway. We talked about how to conserve our time and energy for those things, for the children's sake and for our own. That was what Emer wanted, what we both wanted.

Occasionally people would ask, 'How do you do it?' But what choice did we have? This was our life, our reality, our family. We just had to adjust and keep going. There is no profundity in it. You still have to get up the next day, no matter what has happened. The worst happens, and you get no extra gift of resilience. You just carry on as best you can.

CHAPTER ELEVEN
Getting on with Life
2013

EMER'S INDUCTION THERAPY (INITIAL chemotherapy received before her stem cell transplant) was successful in getting her myeloma under some control. After six months, her paraprotein had dropped significantly. Paraprotein is an abnormal protein produced by myeloma, something that can be monitored as a biomarker to track the disease course and the response to treatment. That drop gave us real hope.

By the early spring of 2013, Emer was healthier and able to do far more, and her pain was under much better control, although she was still on strong painkillers. She was strong enough for a stem cell transplant and so a date was set – immediately after Clodagh's confirmation.

When I look at photos from that confirmation, I can see how well Emer looked then, even though she was starting to lose her hair from the induction therapy. In preparation for the transplant, she was given drugs to stimulate the release of stem cells from the bone marrow and into the bloodstream. From there, they were harvested in a process called apheresis, which is a lot like giving a unit of blood but over a period of hours. The stem cells were then frozen and ready to be reintroduced to her bloodstream as the 'transplant'.

Emer was sensitive about hair loss. I don't think she was unusual in that. I believe that much of her sense of self and identity were bound up, not exactly in the way she looked, because that makes it sound as though she was vain, which she wasn't, but in her physical appearance. Or maybe I should say the physicality of her appearance? I knew that her hair, which was beautiful – very dark and shiny – was important to her. As was the feeling that she looked familiar to the children. Losing her hair was a visible, outward sign of the disease and treatment, and therefore a constant, immediate reminder. But she was obviously keen for the transplant to happen. This was her best hope of remission.

Shortly before going into hospital, she went with Orla, her sister, to Roches in Kimmage to be fitted for a wig. She shaved the remainder of her now very thin hair, and switched to wearing the wig. Orla was a vital support to her in that very difficult part of a journey that so many women have to face.

The day after Clodagh's confirmation in mid-March 2013, Emer was admitted to St James's Hospital, into Burkitt's Ward, the bone marrow transplant unit. She said goodbye to the children before they went to school. That was very difficult for Emer, knowing she wouldn't see them for a month, and knowing she had a difficult few weeks ahead. But she was investing in her treatment, her future and doing everything she could to be available for them. She was very positive about that.

In the four weeks that Emer was in the hospital, we secretly transformed the garden. This was a surprise the children and I had dreamed up for when she came home. I had seen a piece in one of the weekend newspaper supplements about a landscape gardener, Deirdre Prince, that gave me the idea. I telephoned Deirdre, who was instantly engaged by the idea. She surveyed the garden before Emer went into St James's and agreed a plan with me which she committed to complete in a very tight time schedule before Emer came home. I was also having the house painted from top to bottom. With Emer's illness, that kind of disruption was not really possible, but now we had the opportunity.

Late on the day when Emer was admitted for the stem cell transplant, I stood in the back garden. The work had begun. It was starting to snow, and the garden had already been pulled apart. I remember the feeling of mild panic: 'What have I done?' As I stood there in the snow looking at the confusion around me, Emer rang to say her eardrum had perforated and that the transplant would be delayed. This was right out of the blue. Emer had no ear pain and no history of ear problems, even as a child. She said she might have to come home for a few days. I had never imagined anything like this happening! There were builders traipsing in and out through the house, the garden was pulled apart and there were ladders everywhere. In the end, the medical team decided to give her intravenous antibiotics, which meant staying in. I was glad Emer didn't get to see the house that day!

In retrospect, I think this was my way of coping. Keeping myself busy, taking on a lot, maybe too much. I was getting three months' work done in four weeks and managing that was a scramble. My parents came to help me so that I could work, visit Emer, and keep the project going; keep all those bits in the air.

* * *

Ireland held the presidency of the EU in those six months of January to June 2013. That meant I had to host the six-monthly meeting of CMOs from all over Europe. The timing couldn't have been worse. We had a scientific programme and a social programme. In spite of its significance and the preparations that had been put in, I couldn't participate in much of the business of the meeting. Once the opening session had taken place, I had to leave. There simply wasn't time in my day.

Emer received melphalan and then had her harvested stem cells re-infused to become seed for a new marrow. It takes time for that new marrow to develop sufficiently to produce red and white blood cells, and platelets. Therefore, she needed to remain in isolation to limit the risk of serious infection and to have transfusions of red blood cells for haemoglobin and platelets for clotting. Emer's room was sealed and isolated from everyone. She was having multiple blood tests every day. The medical team would appear, gowned and masked, coming in through double doors, then leaving again. It is dehumanising. And an eerie taste of what we would all be doing a few years later during the pandemic.

Emer spent almost five weeks in Burkitt's Ward. Her main contact with the outside world during that time was with me. The children couldn't visit because of the risk of infection. No other visitors were permitted. In that time there were some difficult episodes. While she was at her sickest – with effectively no white cells, a count of 0.0 – and totally dependent on the transfusions, on a few occasions she developed a temperature, a sign of possible infection. Infection represents a major illness for someone with no white cells to help fight it. That meant she had to be treated with broad-spectrum heavy-duty antibiotics.

One morning I visited Emer on my way to work. There was no one at the nurses' station and no one in the room with Emer. That in itself wasn't unusual. The nurses would often be in rooms with other patients as this was a ward of very sick and vulnerable people. But this particular morning I found Emer unwell and confused. I had never seen her like that before. She was speaking incoherently and didn't seem to know me or where she was. She had a temperature. I was frightened by this and worried about sepsis. I pushed the call button, and a short time later a nurse appeared. I said something like, 'Thank goodness you're here.' The nurse's response was to tell me to 'calm down'.

I still remember how deeply upset I was. In general, the nursing staff were really fantastic. I don't think I had ever met that particular nurse before, and I didn't see her again. But I still remember that response – at a moment of such intense vulnerability, when I was so worried, and Emer so sick. I was reacting in an entirely human way, not a medical way. I was really concerned, and her response was dismissive. That sticks out in my mind as an unpleasant memory. I still wonder if I should have done something – said something – but at that moment, I was too concerned about Emer to really focus on that. But it has remained with me. A small example of the way in which the patient's or loved one's experience can suddenly become an unpleasant, dehumanising one.

Thankfully, Emer received excellent care and she started to improve. Her white cell and platelet counts were up. She no longer needed transfusions. And her paraprotein levels came back down to not-detectable levels. This was a cause for real hope. Some people can remain in this state for long periods with no return of a paraprotein 'signal', meaning they effectively stay in remission. The damage to Emer's skeleton would remain, which left her with pain and physical limitations, but these biomarkers showed there was no new activity.

This is where we wanted to be. It had taken seven or eight months of extensive treatment under the direction of Prof Paul Browne to get us here. We were so full of gratitude and hope.

During the last week or so, when her white cells had recovered, she was allowed to go out on walks along the corridors of St James's Hospital. Its long corridors are a great place to build up strength and stamina in preparation for a return home. Clodagh would sometimes come in with me then, and the three of us would have coffee in the coffee dock. Other than Emer being in a dressing gown, this all felt normal. We were so optimistic. We were on the pathway for her to come home. And for Emer to see the new garden.

In truth, we were not sure how she would react. The garden looked amazing but very different. Clodagh, Ronan and I were really excited about this. We felt it would give her a boost. So long as she liked the design. It was mid-April by the time she came home. The new garden was in spring bloom. Emer loved it! The weather was good in Dublin in the summer of 2013 so, whenever she could, Emer would sit on the bench at the end of the garden, in a sheltered spot that gets the sun. Those were wonderful days filled with hope. The disease was in remission and she had stopped all medication.

* * *

That summer, we got to Ballybunion, which is where Emer was always happiest. Her family had holidayed there for three weeks every summer ever since she was a small child. It was a wonderful, long-standing tradition, one that we adopted with our family. We would join Emer's parents every year from when Clodagh was born. The annual Feely Ballybunion trip expanded to include Emer's siblings and their children as they were born over the coming years. We would spend every dry day and a few rainy ones sitting in a circle on the beach. Happy times.

And for about a year, although Emer continued to deal with fatigue and residual pains, she had no new symptoms. Symptom-free control is the aim with myeloma. Steroids had caused her to gain a little weight, and she had by now lost that. She bought herself a completely new wardrobe of clothes. Her hair grew back. She felt really good about herself, and positive about life and the future.

Sadly, that bright phase lasted only a short period of time.

* * *

I can still remember Emer ringing me to tell me her paraprotein levels had gone up. I was cycling home from work one evening with no sense that bad news was around the corner. It was a year or so after the transplant, and she was still having her paraprotein checked regularly. She got such a boost each time the results were good. For just over a year they were. And then they weren't.

We had to reinstitute chemotherapy. That then became the norm and she never came off chemotherapy until shortly before she died. But she incorporated it into her life. She continued to work. On her way to work in Dr Steevens' Hospital she would stop at St James's Hospital, have an infusion of chemo-therapy, then go on to work. Sometimes she'd need a day off, or to work from home, and her colleagues were very under-standing and accommodating. They focused on enabling her to do what she could.

Emer was adamant that she wanted to be given challenging work. She didn't want to feel in any sense that work was being diverted away from her because she wasn't deemed to be well enough. I think that was a part of her identity, and valuable confirmation of her wellness at a point in time. For Clodagh and Ronan too, it was reassuring for them to see life going on as 'normal', and see that Emer was able to be out and about and doing what she had always done. Ultimately, though, it became a greater challenge. She had too many symptoms, and the disease was taking too much of a toll. In 2017 she had to retire on disability grounds.

* * *

Emer's medication regime was constantly evolving. One of the drugs she started on was initially an infusion to be given over hours in the day ward of the hospital. Over time this was replaced by an injection that could be given subcutaneously, something that took a matter of minutes instead of hours on a drip. Later again, a 'cousin' of that drug was developed that could be taken orally, so she didn't have to go into hospital to take it. These differences in drugs make a big impact on patients' lives, and the lives of their families.

She experienced many side effects, including nausea and peripheral neuropathy, meaning she lost feeling in her legs and feet. She still had a lot of pain associated with the new lesions. But she was on pain medication and this was reasonably well managed. I know the pain was with her nearly constantly, draining her energy and resources. But at that time, there was really nothing in her life that was important to her that she could not do.

At this time, even though the disease had come back, we were still at the point where there were lots of options should the drugs she was on become ineffective. And that was a good place to be. We didn't by any means feel we were running out of road. Quite the contrary. The advances made for blood cancers generally in the last decade have been enormous, and Emer benefited from that. In the latter half of her illness, she was taking two anti-myeloma drugs that hadn't even been licensed when she was diagnosed.

She had great faith in the public service and the treatment she was getting at St James's Hospital. She felt she owed it to the children, however, to be sure there wasn't something available in, say, the USA that could have benefited her. Prof Paul Browne was very generous about this. Some doctors don't respond well to such requests, but Paul was the opposite. He found the appropriate people for her to talk to in the USA;

people involved in research at the Dana-Farber Cancer Institute in Boston, a world leader in the field. We decided to make the trip and for it to be a family holiday.

Around Hallowe'en of 2015, the four of us flew to Boston and spent four days there, of which about half a day was spent going to see Professor Paul Richardson at the Dana-Farber Institute. He was very involved in research on myeloma. There were no silver bullets – we knew that. Professor Richardson agreed that there were options in terms of other drugs, and these were all available for Emer in Ireland if required. That brought her a sense of reassurance and peace.

After Boston, we hired a car and drove to Manhattan through the New England colour. We stayed in Times Square, saw all the sights, and went out to Jersey Gardens, one of these enormous outlet shopping centres, where I was happy to be the bag carrier for the day. It was a once-in-a-lifetime holiday with the children. And Emer took something extra from it – the certainty that she was doing absolutely everything she could. That was really important for her.

CHAPTER TWELVE
CervicalCheck: First Knowledge

BY 2018 I HAD been CMO for ten years. In that time, I had led the introduction of Healthy Ireland and a number of public health policies relating to obesity, physical activity, alcohol, tobacco and sexual health. I had dealt with the dioxin crisis, swine flu, and patient safety issues such as the use of vaginal mesh in surgery and gynaecology and the response to the congenital impact of the use of sodium valproate as a treatment during pregnancy for illnesses such as epilepsy, bipolar illness and chronic pain. My division had also developed legislation prohibiting female genital mutilation and the 2013 Protection of Life During Pregnancy Act, which allowed for termination of pregnancy to protect the life of the mother. In 2018 we were also time-intensively engaged in the work on repealing the Eighth Amendment of the Constitution and preparing the proposed legislation and service developments.

In all that time, nothing had come close to the impact related to the CervicalCheck crisis. CervicalCheck was a perfect storm. A blend of complicated, often specialised, information, a complex unrolling of events, passionate and articulate advocates, and heart-breaking personal stories.

My concern from the outset was that this would have an undue negative impact on the healthcare system and on people's confidence in screening in particular. I was not the only one. From the very beginning, there was confusion, misinformation and disinformation. Given this and also how intense a time this was for the women affected, and their families and friends, I think it is important that I give my account of what happened.

In the early 2000s, as one of the Department of Health's deputy CMOs, I had been deeply involved in cancer policy and service improvement. In those days, the health service had a breast cancer screening programme, not yet fully national in scope, and had no state-organised cervical cancer screening programme.

At the time, it was well established through health research and evidence that a country could not expect to make improvements on cervical cancer mortality at the population level without organising a screening programme based on good public health principles. Any such screening programme should be population-based, have a high uptake, operate good call-and-recall, use expert labs with appropriate activity levels, and have good referral arrangements for women whose smears required follow-up with colposcopy. This whole system should be underpinned by end-to-end quality assurance.

Ireland was late in setting up a national cervical cancer screening programme compared with some other countries. The UK began a pap-based smear programme in 1964 – named after the Greek doctor, George Papanicolaou, who developed it – and established the NHS-organised population-based screening programme in 1988.

In the mid-2000s, women in Ireland were having pap smears on an individual basis rather than a population basis. In other words, the procedure might be suggested by their GP or gynae-cologist or an opportunity might arise in clinics, but there was no state-organised programme that was directed at ensuring all women had access to a national screening service to which they would be invited to participate in at the right time, without needing medical referral or financial means to do so. There were two main problems with this pre-existing ad hoc approach.

While the numbers being screened were substantial for the size of the population (we knew the number of smears received by Irish laboratories was 218,000 in 2001 and we estimated that this would have increased further to perhaps as many as 300,000 smears per annum), the structure of the system and the demographic of the people being screened were not adequate. We needed a structured system with the ability to call and recall patients as required, with cytology, which is the process of examining smears on a slide with a microscope, being carried out in accredited laboratories and the process properly audited.

The second issue was that a pattern had emerged that smear tests were apparently being carried out too frequently on some women, and not at all on other women. The sad truth is that social disadvantage is a risk factor for cervical cancer. Meaning that hard-to-reach groups – those who weren't coming forward as frequently – were statistically the ones most likely to get cervical cancer. It was, therefore, important that a screening programme be easily available for this vulnerable section of the population and that uptake be monitored to ensure they were accessing it.

* * *

Prior to the establishment of CervicalCheck, we had more than a dozen laboratories in Ireland processing pap smear tests, only five of which were processing in excess of the recommended minimum of 15,000 smears per year. The bigger Irish laborat-ories collectively carried out the great majority of the smears, but there were many smaller ones processing far less than international norms and routinely recommended volumes. I can even recall there were reports of pathologists reading slides at domestic kitchen tables. We knew that women deserved a much better-organised service at a national level.

Women who were having smears carried out before the establishment of the national screening programme were entitled to believe and to expect they were getting an appropriate service, but the truth was that there was a lot of room for improvement.

As deputy CMO I had been able to work on some of the initial arrangements to nationalise the programme. Phase one of the Irish Cervical Screening Programme (ICSP) had already been established and was being delivered through the Mid-Western Health Board. We set about expanding this, and getting the funding in place to bring it to national level.

There were plenty of key people involved, one of whom was Dr Grainne Flannelly. She had come back to Ireland in the early 2000s, having been a gynaecologist in the UK, and was a passionate advocate for the cervical screening programme. Grainne came to meet with Minister for Health Mary Harney, my colleagues and I, and spoke about her time in the UK. She had only rarely seen the late presentations of cervical cancer that we were seeing in Ireland at the time. She talked about young women with advanced stage three and four presentations of cervical cancer, how traumatic their treatment was at these stages, and how poor the survival rates. These were very often women with young children. Grainne explained that such cases were rare in the UK, and all too common in Ireland. She was articulate and passionate, and I have no doubt played a pivotal role in generating political commitment to the programme. She certainly made an impression on Mary Harney and on me. Grainne went on to become the clinical director of our national screening programme. CervicalCheck began in 2008, at a time of national and global economic crisis. And yet Mary Harney found money to prioritise this programme, when so many other projects were being closed down because there simply weren't resources to keep them going.

At the time, the BreastCheck programme was managed by an independent national agency. Tony O'Brien, who went on to head up the HSE, was the CEO. The HSE took on responsibility for CervicalCheck and BreastCheck as the National Cancer Screening Service (NCSS), which in turn was part of the wider National Cancer Control Programme. In around 2014, the National Health and Wellbeing Programme of the HSE took responsibility for running the NCSS, alongside other population-based programmes such as immunisation.

As part of the establishment of CervicalCheck, cytology was outsourced by the programme to laboratories in the USA that had the capacity to manage this. Without their capacity a national programme would not have been possible. At the time, many women had been experiencing very long delays in receiving their smear reports.

The international evidence was clear: a national screening programme could reduce the incidence of cervical cancer, and ultimately reduce mortality. Unlike breast screening, which picks up early cancer, the cytology-based screening programme for cervical cancer is designed to pick up abnormalities, where possible, before a cancer emerges. And so we wanted to introduce this as part of the cancer strategy.

Cervical cancer develops in the cells of the cervix, which is the lower part of the uterus that connects to the vagina. Human papillomavirus (HPV) infections are the main cause of cervical cancer. HPV infections are common, and most people who have them do not experience any symptoms. While there are more than a hundred types of HPV, only some cause cancer. These types include HPV-16 and HPV-18, which are responsible for around 70 per cent of all cases of cervical cancer.

At the outset, we knew that there are limitations to any screening service. The reality is that not every person who has the abnormality or syndrome being screened for will be found. Thus, someone could be screened and provided with a 'nothing to be found' result, and then subsequently develop a cancer. That's called a 'false negative' finding. Furthermore, the programme will inevitably pick up people who do not in fact have the abnormality or syndrome but are then subjected to further diagnostic interventions and treatments. That's known as a 'false positive'. This point is readily understood and accepted by most people when it is explained clearly to them.

People might reasonably ask why we have these national screening programmes if they are imperfect systems that some-times produce false assessments. In public health terms, you make sure that screening programmes are only established at the population level when the benefits from picking up enough cases that can then be prevented or treated outweigh the down-sides of some people unfortunately being missed (false negatives) by an imperfect screening test and some others being harmed by investigations and treatments they would not have had had they not been falsely identified (false positives). It is crucial that this point is understood – but very often it is not. Screening tests are not diagnostic tests. Even if you receive an abnormal screening test result you still need to be referred for a diagnosis, and no test is perfect.

I fully recognise and empathise with any woman who discovers she has cervical cancer after previously receiving a false negative on her screening, and who therefore may have missed a chance for earlier detection of an abnormality, and the subsequent impact this has on her and her family. The harsh truth is that it is never possible to eliminate that risk from a cervical screening programme. Despite the understandable instinct to identify a particular cause or reason to blame, a false negative on a screening programme is not an automatic or prima facie evidence of negligence. While, unfortunately, human error or negligence can undoubtedly occur, what has emerged post-CervicalCheck is a widespread belief that every false negative is negligent.

That incorrect belief among some people arises from misunderstandings about a new quality assurance initiative that CervicalCheck and the HSE decided to introduce: a post-cancer diagnosis retrospective audit.

* * *

CervicalCheck had strong quality assurance built into its screening programme. Many programmes in other European countries do not have such arrangements. A report from the European Commission in 2017 showed that 16 European countries had a dedicated quality assurance team for cervical screening, while 11 did not. To the credit of the leadership of the Irish NCSS, they put these quality assurance arrangements in place.

One such arrangement was the post-cancer diagnosis retrospective audit. In simple terms, this means that every time a diagnosis of cervical cancer was made, the programme wanted to determine, first, whether the woman had been screened by it and, second, if and why an opportunity, however small, to prevent that cancer had been missed. This was to allow lessons to be learned and further improvements to be made to the programme for the benefit of women who were to be screened in the future.

As managers of the CervicalCheck screening programme, those with responsibility in the HSE had regular engagements with the Department of Health, including some of my staff and colleagues in other parts of the Department. They would periodically tell us what was happening, so that I had a general sense of the running of the CervicalCheck programme, as one component of all public health-related programmes run by the HSE. In 2016, the HSE informed us that the NCSS was preparing to disclose findings to women of their post-cancer diagnosis retrospective audit in which there was a different ('discordant') finding from an earlier screening report. If I had any objection in principle to such a disclosure, that was the time I would have voiced it. I had no such objection.

There were a number of considerations they had to take into account when introducing a policy of disclosing such findings to women. The first was whether they should give the patient the option of receiving the results of a retrospective audit of their screening slide. The UK's experience showed that when given the option, very often the patient declined. Having already been diagnosed with cancer, they were now receiving, or had received, or had successfully completed, treatment for it. They saw little value in being told of a re-examination of their screening slides by someone who now knew they had cancer and was potentially biased as a result that might show that there may have been new or different cytological findings than those previously reported. Other women in the UK had indicated they did want to know their result from the audit.

In most countries in the world, there is no option to be informed of false negative test results identified through retrospective audits of diagnosed cancers. Ireland is one of the few countries where this is possible. Canada has legislative prohibition on such audit disclosure in most provinces. The Netherlands and Denmark also have legislation that prevents the results of an audit being disclosed. The information is deliberately not given back to patients. This is because it's being collected to improve the service for future users as opposed to being an integral part of the system of care for an individual.

From the patient's perspective, this latter point is worth explaining further. I know and understand the personal impact that a diagnosis of life-threatening cancer can have on the lives of women and men, at whatever stage they learn about it. The provision of screening services to detect the possibility of cervical cancer developing, and providing necessary treatments, is part of any modern healthcare system. Monitoring and learning about how those screening services can be improved for patients is an essential part of providing them. From a strict quality assurance point of view, the diagnosis of cervical cancer in an individual patient who had previously been through the screening programme is primarily an opportunity to look back to determine if any deficits or weaknesses can be identified, addressed and rectified. This is so that other patients may benefit from continuously improving training, processes and standards.

By their very nature, the findings of such an audit cannot make any difference to the diagnosis and treatment planning for an individual patient because it is auditing patients who were already diagnosed with cancer.

A second consideration, as part of the planning process to set up the audit, was for the CervicalCheck programme to make arrangements whereby, should any issues arise from individual cases, there would be proper and effective communication to the patient via medical professionals. As a responsible programme, they also had to consider how they would best handle a situation where a case, following the planned disclosure, received media attention, and any legal issues that might arise. Their concern, rightly, was for the potential impact on public confidence in the programme, which could lead to reduced uptake of the programme, thereby risking the health and lives of other women.

This kind of contingency planning and working through potential scenarios and 'what-ifs' around the introduction of the post-cancer diagnosis retrospective audit and informing patients of possible results was part and parcel of good management. Population-based programmes around the world make similar provisions and contingency plans. That's how we in the Department of Health understood it: as a good-quality assurance development being put together by the Cervical Screening Programme with the HSE.

The NCSS decided that it would provide discordant audit results to individual patients. It commenced doing so in 2016, reporting the findings to individual clinicians of the women concerned. What no one knew until 2018 was that the findings of the post-cancer diagnosis retrospective audit were never actually given to the majority of the women concerned. I only discovered that when a team of us conducted a detailed chart review over a weekend in late April 2018. That review only happened the day after the verdict was given in the court case taken by the late Vicky Phelan.

* * *

On the morning of Thursday 26 April 2018, someone drew my attention to reports of a court case relating to CervicalCheck which had come to media attention. That was my first hint of what was coming. Later that morning, I ran into a senior colleague who raised it with me in corridor conversation, asking if I had heard anything about it. I said I had some general awareness but not much more than that.

I was having a late sandwich that same day in a nearby coffee shop with another colleague who was a senior person in the department. As we sat, she received a call from the minister, Simon Harris, who said he wanted to immediately announce an investigation led by the HSE into this issue, which had been reported on the lunchtime news.

I was thinking, 'We don't even know what this is about. We have nothing to go on apart from reports in the media, and he wants to announce an investigation?' So I asked my colleague if I could speak to him. I took the phone and went outside into the street.

The minister was insisting, 'We have to investigate.' We had no real idea, as yet, what had actually happened. My feeling was that we had to be very cautious not to do anything rash that would later cause harm to the screening programme. I asked him, 'Can you give me a bit of time to work out what this is about, so that we can specify the terms of any investigation?' But no. He absolutely wanted to announce publicly that action was being taken that very afternoon.

I knew Simon Harris reasonably well at this point and was used to dealing with him. I realised he was not for turning on this matter and was not minded to take my advice. I went back to my office and took what was an unusual step for me. I felt I had no option but to put my thoughts in writing. I wrote an email asking that he hold off an announcement for now on the basis of this case at least until we could establish some preliminary facts – pretty much what I had said to him earlier on the telephone – and that not to do so risked undue reputational harm for the screening service.

Instead, I suggested, he could 'state that you have asked me to provide a report on the matter, including whether further actions or steps are required'. My thinking behind this email was 'Don't jump into this; walk in slowly, so when you do announce something, it will be the right thing, will be robust and will stand up to scrutiny.' All the experience I had had previously – sometimes difficult experience – told me this was the right way to proceed.

In particular, I was thinking of a harrowing situation I had been involved with in relation to neonatal deaths in Portlaoise.

That was a situation that emerged in 2014. A *Prime Time Investigates* report in late January alleged that four otherwise healthy babies had died during labour in the Midland Regional Hospital in Portlaoise as a result of hospital errors. The programme specifically alleged that investigations into these deaths, which had occurred over a period of time, had led to findings that were not implemented and which could have prevented later deaths. That immediately raised a serious question, which required a decisive response.

As a first step, Minister Reilly and I travelled to Portlaoise on the Sunday after the public revelation and met the parents of each of the four babies in succession. This took many hours and made an enormous impression on both of us. I think it strengthened the minister's resolve to approach the matter quickly but methodically. There were very serious issues in question which had potential implications for obstetric services throughout the country.

As a doctor, Minister Reilly had the same concerns that I did. He asked me to go immediately to Portlaoise Hospital to find out what was going on and report back to him so we could establish what further actions might be necessary. He gave me three or four weeks in which to do this, a very short time frame.

I responded immediately and assembled a small team of people I trusted and had high regard for, led by Kathleen MacLellan, who later went on to have the distinction of being appointed to direct the first National Patient Safety Office, the creation of which was an ultimate consequence of the events in Portlaoise. We met the families again, visited the hospital a number of times and met the relevant staff. We completed a report to the minister in two and a half weeks. He published it immediately.

The report was comprehensive and didn't pull any punches. The findings were that each of the four deaths had been previously separately investigated, wholly or in part by the hospital, but in each case, these investigations were followed by a failure to fully and verifiably implement the findings, which then placed other babies at risk. We recommended that a detailed investigation by HIQA (the Health Information and Quality Authority) should follow, and Minister Reilly ordered it.

We concluded that Portlaoise Maternity Unit was not a safe service and therefore should not continue to run itself. We took steps to address that, recommending that the Coombe Hospital manage operations there while the necessary changes were made. This was planned and carried out in accordance with the appropriate prioritisation of patient safety risk, something that absolutely must inform decisions at a time like that. At the top of that hierarchy is the likelihood of continuing risk. If there is any possibility that a person who is yet to use a particular service is at risk, that is the most pressing concern, and must be acted on quickly. In an extreme case, a temporary service closure might be required.

Next would be something that may have happened historically, but where people may benefit from being identified in case the harm requires further treatment or services. An example of this would be a point source exposure to a blood-borne virus infection; for example a procedure carried out on a patient who was later found to be hepatitis B positive. In such a case, there may be a need to determine if any other patient or staff members have been exposed.

The third tier of priority from a service point of view is a situation in which something harmful has happened to an individual, where there is no reason to believe or suspect that occurrence points up risks for former or future patients. This is not at the same scale as an event which has harmed or risks harming many people. An investigation may be warranted, but without the imperative of the other two categories.

* * *

There was nothing apparent on that Thursday in April from the media report about the court case on CervicalCheck to suggest that disclosures of discordant post-cancer diagnosis audit findings had not taken place for the majority of women. It was important to ascertain the facts. It certainly needed to be understood and acted upon, but there wasn't the urgency that would have arisen from believing other women were at active risk.

Hence my advice for proceeding calmly and rationally was informed by the knowledge that in the post-cancer diagnosis audit such retrospective information is not likely to be time-sensitive in the way that clinical information is. Three days later, on the Sunday evening (as I will come to describe), we had established some key facts about what had actually happened and how many women were potentially involved. These new facts made it clear that we needed a significant investigation – and one that would not be led by, but instead had to be independent of, the HSE. But having first established these facts, we were now in a position to know what the terms of such an investigation needed to be. On that first day, the idea of 'an investigation led by the HSE' – without any specific question upon which to base an investigation – seemed rash.

As far as I was aware, when I spoke with the minister, he had no more information than I did. I sent the email urging him to take a little bit of time before making a media announce-ment, but he came back and said he was going ahead. At that, I emailed again, saying 'I am strongly advising you not to proceed.' But there was no stopping him.

He announced an investigation, to be undertaken by Tony O'Brien and the HSE. By lunchtime the next day, Friday 27 April, we had already learned enough to know that his proposal was inadequate and so it never proceeded. Some subsequent media reporting of my actions led to headlines saying I tried to block the Scally investigation, using my emails to the minister on the first day as evidence for this. That is and was completely false and utterly at variance with the facts. The reality was completely different: what I initially proposed in that email to the minister should happen is exactly what did happen – an initial assessment to get as many facts as possible to determine the scope of the problem (which we had completed by the Sunday evening), and then setting the terms of an independent investigation to be carried out in more depth, which was ultimately to be carried out by an appropriate person, i.e. Gabriel Scally, who was recommended by me.

On that Friday, 27 April, we had a better understanding of Vicky Phelan's case. It had become clear that what was alleged was that information relating to a post-cancer diagnosis retrospective audit that was to have been passed back to her had not been. However, there were also reports of a 'gagging order', that she and her legal team made reference to, and I did not understand what that was or why it was in place or who had asked for it.

What I heard being alleged was that whoever did the post-cancer diagnosis retrospective audit had a different view of some of the smears that had been taken before the diagnosis of cancer. This was not anything unusual to find in the context of a later cervical cancer diagnosis. Reading cervical smear slides is highly skilled work, and a degree of interpretation is required. Therefore, it was common that a retrospective reading of slides of a person known to have developed cervical cancer, which had been deemed clear at one point in time, might later report them as abnormal.

Nothing so far relating to this case, clinically speaking, rang alarm bells for me. But at least now we had a question: 'What exactly is the state of play with the post-cancer diagnosis retrospective audit?'

In a meeting with the minister and the secretary general, which took place around Friday lunchtime in the minister's office in Leinster House, I told the minister that I would go up to the CervicalCheck offices on Parnell Street and that I wouldn't leave until I found out what was going on.

By 4pm on Friday, I had assembled a team of colleagues for the purpose from the HSE and the Department of Health and was headed for Parnell Street to meet the CervicalCheck top management team. We set about understanding exactly what had been happening with the audit and the practice of disclosure to women of discordant findings from it. I made it clear that we were going to have to find a way to go through every chart from every hospital, every file of every woman diagnosed with cervical cancer where there was a reported discordance in a smear result prior to her diagnosis. We were going to have to find out if there had been a documented disclosure discussion of these findings with each of those women. And we were going to have to do that as fast as possible.

Somebody said at one point, 'It's half-five on a Friday evening, everyone in the hospitals around the country will be going home shortly.' To which my response was, 'Tough luck.' We had no choice. This had to be done. Immediately. That was my determination,

On that Friday evening, we had no idea where the 'known facts' would take us. Once we started to pull that thread, we couldn't know what it might be connected to. But as far as I was concerned the thread needed to be pulled.

CHAPTER THIRTEEN

CervicalCheck: Second Stage

WE WERE EFFECTIVELY CAMPED out in Parnell Street at the NCSS headquarters for the entire weekend. Over the course of those two days, teams of people in the HSE were dispatched to physically go into chart rooms of hospitals across the country, and pull charts of women diagnosed with cervical cancer. These were then examined by clinicians, to ensure that these cases had been diagnosed with cervical cancer and had a prior history of screening at least once with CervicalCheck. The charts were examined to determine if there was a discordant report from a post-cancer diagnosis retrospective audit and if there was evidence of it having been disclosed to the woman. All that information was recorded, and bit by bit we built up a clear picture of what had happened.

The charts were chosen according to two different databases. The first was women who had been through the screening programme and were on the CervicalCheck database. The second was women with cervical cancer in the National Cancer Registry database. The two didn't always match. There were women who had been picked up by the cancer registry programme who didn't have a screening history. Between 2008 and 2018, 3310 cervical cancer cases were recorded by the

National Cancer Registry; 1482 (44.8 per cent) had been screened and subsequently were diagnosed with cervical cancer.

These had to be reconciled in order to find out how many women might potentially not have had discordant post-cancer diagnosis retrospective audit findings disclosed so we could understand whether the issue was confined to the one case now in the courts, or if it was more extensive than that.

This process was largely complete by Sunday afternoon and we had an idea of the number of women involved. That number finally settled at 221 women where the audit and the earlier findings were at variance with one another. (It wasn't 221 that day – I recall it was 209. We identified most but not all the affected women in that initial weekend review.)

Teams in the individual hospitals were able to go through the charts and find that in around 75 per cent of these cases, there was no evidence documented of a disclosure having taken place. So for at least three-quarters of these women there was no evidence a disclosure had been made. And therefore we had to presume that the disclosure had not happened.

Now we knew for certain, for the first time, that this was a systemic problem. CervicalCheck had a policy to disclose this information, and had not done so. While this failure did not in any way affect the women's treatment and outcomes, it was a breach of an important commitment that had been given.

Something I didn't know at the time but discovered later was that, as a community, the colposcopists and gynaecologists had never bought into the idea of post-cancer diagnosis retrospective disclosure. These people were later heavily criticised as misogynists and were lambasted in public. Their point was, they had never signed up to this. They had never thought it was a good idea, and had been very clear about that from the start. Their belief was that it couldn't help the women involved, and might indeed cause more, avoidable, distress.

So what happened was that information gleaned from the post-cancer diagnosis retrospective audit was being posted out to individual consultants, some of whom didn't feed that information back to the women concerned. Many of these women would have completed early and effective treatment in the years prior and had in effect been cured and discharged from the service of the consultant who was now expected to feed this information back to them. In many cases the information was filed in patient charts, but women were not told about it.

This was a breach of trust. That's what we needed to deal with.

*   *   *

Meanwhile, across the course of that weekend, the media and political storm continued unabated. At some stage on the Saturday afternoon, I received a phone call to advise me that the minister had done a pre-recorded interview for that evening's *Six One News*. The caller stated that, 'I think the minister has gone too far.' I asked what that meant and was informed that he may have said something which the caller couldn't recall precisely, that could make Grainne Flannery's position untenable. I called Stephen Mulvaney to alert him as acting CEO of the HSE (Tony O'Brien was away).

That night Grainne Flannery resigned. That really coloured the medical profession's response to all of this, because it instilled fear. You couldn't get anyone to take any kind of responsibility after that. As far as due process and natural justice was concerned, this felt wrong to me. The process of investigation hadn't really begun, and yet Grainne was placed in a position where she believed she had no choice but to announce her resignation. I didn't hear strong voices of support coming out for her from the leadership or board of the HSE in spite of all she had done for women's health.

My belief was that those of us who had leadership positions within the professions needed to face this head on, no matter how peripheral our responsibility. We had a duty to step up and respond to the public's need to be informed. We needed to do our best to restore trust and confidence in the screening programme, while remaining conscious of the impact to these individual women and the need for an investigation to take place. But once Grainne went, it was very difficult to make that point of view stick. I cannot recall any issue where there was such widespread fear on the part of the medical profession and its key members.

The following evening, Sunday 29 April, I briefed the minister on what my team's initial chart review had revealed about the extent and scope of the issue, and the likely terms of reference that would be required for an investigation to be led independently by an external professional. The minister was grateful for the updated information and agreed with the need for a major independent investigation.

* * *

The following week, on Tuesday 1 May as I recall, I organised a press conference because I was convinced that with questions to be answered, the right thing to do for those who held senior leadership positions was to give answers as best we could. At that conference were myself, Jerome Coffey (director of the Cancer Control Programme), Colm Henry (chief clinical officer at the HSE), Donal Brennan (professor of obstetrics and gynaecology at UCD) and Kathleen McLellan (director of the National Patient Safety Office).

We conducted the press conference in the College of Physicians in an atmosphere that I have never seen before or since. By then it was clear that there was systemic, widespread non-disclosure to patients of the screening programme, and the press were hostile. No longer impartial. No longer analytical. There were very few voices of reason. This was in stark contrast to the measured response of the Swedish media to reports published in 2020 of increased numbers of women diagnosed with cervical cancer following a normal smear report between 2008 and 2015 in that country.

The day after the press conference, the HSE and the Department attended a meeting of the Public Accounts Committee. That morning, on *Morning Ireland*, there had been another significant event – Emma Mhic Mhathúna had come forward to tell her own harrowing story. She was a young mother of five children, with a late-stage diagnosis of cervical cancer. I recall one Public Accounts Committee member shouting at Tony O'Brien, whom I was seated beside, that he had 'blood on his hands'.

In the course of that morning, answering the questions of the committee, Tony O'Brien made reference to a document from 2016 about HSE planning for the introduction of the audit. I would have seen copies of these notes at the time. The documents made reference to legal views that would be sought by the HSE in advance of the audit starting. The clear context was the CervicalCheck programme being rightly concerned with creating the proper conditions and preparations for disclosure to patients of the findings of the post-cancer diagnosis retrospective audit.

The committee asked if he could produce the documents and they were duly published that afternoon by the HSE. However, once published, two things became conflated: the recent knowledge that there was a practice of widespread non-disclosure of post-cancer diagnosis retrospective audit findings; and the fact

118

that the HSE was getting legal and communications advice in order to facilitate effective implementation of the CervicalCheck policy to openly disclose findings of post-cancer diagnosis retrospective audit. These were two completely different things. But the distinction was entirely lost in the public discourse.

The conclusion was widely and wrongly drawn that, contrary to CervicalCheck policy, women would routinely or frequently have post-cancer diagnosis retrospective audit findings withheld, and that this was known by people in 2016. In reality, no one outside the CervicalCheck programme knew that until April 2018, as a result of the chart review that I and others carried out after Vicky Phelan's case came to light.

* * *

At this stage, a proper response clearly needed to be put in place. We needed a process that was capable of finding answers to all the questions that had been raised. That led to the Scally Report and an audit by the Royal College of Obstetrics and Gynaecology (RCOG) in the UK.

The terms of reference for each of these reports were drawn up by a very small group of top-level officials in the Department of Health, including me. I knew Gabriel Scally, having met him a few times at international meetings. Born in Belfast, he had trained in Northern Ireland, and worked mostly in the UK, where, as well as roles in public health, he had also led several inquiries into serious NHS clinical failures. Some of his career had been spent in Northern Ireland – he had been director of public health for the Eastern Health and Social Services Board – meaning he understood Ireland, which was important, but he wasn't from a particular hospital, or with an existing set of allegiances, which was also important.

I rang Gabriel on a Saturday morning (5 May 2018) and asked if he would agree to carrying out this review. He did. He reviewed the process from end to end, publishing his report in September 2018. He made important findings and recommendations which have been the subject of a significant implementation programme. As a result there have been major improvements made not only to cervical screening but to the health system generally.

Scally needed to walk a very difficult line. He needed to have the trust and confidence of the women and families concerned. But that didn't mean just telling them what they wanted to hear. He needed to relate his findings to the facts, which he did. And he certainly didn't pull his punches.

Meanwhile, the RCOG in London carried out the technical review, along with the British Association for Cytology and Colposcopy (BACCP). To all intent and purposes, it was an audit of the original audit. They examined the slides to assess the extent of any discordance with the earlier findings in the post-cancer diagnosis retrospective audit and the original assessments carried out by CervicalCheck. The RCOG/BACCP review found no evidence that the screening programme had performed to a standard below that expected for a population-based programme for cervical cytology.

The evidence of these reviews is that the screening programme did what it was intended to do. Which was to perform at a population level, to contribute to a reduction of incidence and thereby to reduce the risk of mortality from cervical cancer.

What it did not do was deliver on the commitment in its own policy to openly disclose findings of post-cancer diagnosis retrospective audits to the women concerned. That should not have happened. The breach of trust and resultant damage to public confidence in the service could have been avoided.

* * *

I met Vicky Phelan only once, in May or June 2018, at a meeting involving other patient representatives, the Irish Cancer Society and senior officials from the Department of Health and the HSE. It took place in the Westin Hotel near the Department of Health. I felt sympathy for her as a young mother of young children, who was dying. I could relate to this all too well. I could understand what her family must have been going through. I was impressed at how she gave time and energy to advocate for improvement of cervical screening services in spite of the physical and psychological impact of her illness. That was what I felt, above anything else, in relation to her.

I came to know Emma Mhic Mhathúna better – and of course felt the same sympathy for her as a mother of young children who was dying from advanced cervical cancer. I was initially asked to speak to her following a meeting she had with President Higgins. That request came from senior staff in Áras an Uachtaráin, as Emma had been asking them about access to medicines and to clinical trials. She and I initially spoke in mid-June 2018 and stayed in close communication until later that summer, when her health began to decline.

I had an opportunity, at her request, to help her access medical and other consultations that she needed. I also helped her with accessing consular assistance when she found herself admitted to hospital in Morocco on a holiday with relatives. She shared my aim to ensure that lessons were learned so that the programme would be protected from unnecessary negative impact. Emma was clear about what she wanted to say and why she was saying it. She was very forthcoming, in our conversations and in the messages and voicemails she sent me, in her criticisms of people she felt did not share her motivation. Mostly, I was impressed with how she spoke about her children and how she wanted to ensure they could be cared for and protected as much as possible from her impending death. I could relate to that very readily.

* * *

The scale of the CervicalCheck controversy unfortunately led to a delay in the introduction of HPV screening. This is a superior screening test for the presence of the HPV virus that causes cervical cancer. When the virus is found, those who are found to have HPV receive more intense monitoring and screening with cervical smears.

The swab is similar, but simpler to perform, and the results are much more reliable. It does not rely on the judgement of a human – a cytologist – to identify subtle abnormalities in cells. In cytology, there is significant scope for two people looking at the same slide to come to different conclusions. This even applies to the same person looking at a slide on different days. The HPV test is an automated test which is not based on human interpretation.

There has been much improvement to CervicalCheck and related services since 2018, thanks to people speaking out and to a wide range of organisations and agencies working together to make the necessary improvements and to painstakingly restore trust. Cervical cancer is unique in that we now have two well-run and highly effective programmes in place to prevent it – screening and vaccination. Through these two prevention programmes we have a real prospect of achieving cervical cancer elimination, meaning a reduction in its incidence to less than 5 per cent of what it would be without those programmes. It is appropriate to recall the leadership of Laura Brennan, someone I did not have an opportunity to meet, in making in the case for HPV immunisation while she was ill and dying from cervical cancer. Many women will avoid development of cervical cancer as a result of this vaccine.

For women under 50, cervical cancer was a major public health risk. There is no other cancer or clinical syndrome where we have two major technologies designed to prevent it. When I think about that, it is truly amazing. It gives me hope for lots of other cancers in the future, and it underlines the value of prevention. It is good to see that HPV vaccination and screening programmes in Ireland are achieving very high uptake by international standards.

The CervicalCheck crisis shows how vital public trust is to the operation of any service and how easily and quickly it can be lost. It shows how difficult it can be to re-establish that trust. In particular, it shows that a breach in trust by a service provider, in this case the failure to honour a commitment to give information to women that was promised to them, can leave people deeply distrustful and vulnerable.

It shows how easily misunderstandings and false beliefs can be established among the public and that once established, they seem to persist, even when the facts show them to be false. It is noteworthy that many times since that crisis, people in leadership positions with respect to screening who have made really impressive efforts to explain these complex issues have been the subject of personal criticism from some quarters.

Two years later, when Covid-19 emerged, the experience of CervicalCheck made me clearer than I ever would otherwise have been about just how central public trust would need to be and that we should do everything in our power to establish, maintain and protect it.

CHAPTER FOURTEEN
The Abortion Referendum

IN THE REFERENDUM ON the Eighth Amendment to the Constitution, which took place on 25 May 2018, two out of every three people voted to repeal Article 40.3.3. It was a momentous day for the country and a day that was a long time coming for those of us involved in the preparation.

At the time many thousands of women each year had no choice but to travel outside the country, mostly to the UK, to have access to a termination of pregnancy. I felt personally that women were being denied access to an important health service. As CMO, I was in a position to influence this. While there may be different perspectives on termination of pregnancy and whether it should be accessible in Ireland, it could not be disputed that the absence of a choice in Ireland was a major public health and patient safety issue.

Having to travel meant, for example, that many women were having terminations later in pregnancy, which meant greater risks; that women did not have continuity of care for complications, such as infection, that arose after their return to Ireland; and that many women feared revealing that they had had a termination of pregnancy to their doctor or health service provider in Ireland.

There are many starting points leading to the referendum for different people involved. For me, the story began in December 2010, by which time I had been CMO for two years. News broke of a court judgment in cases taken by three women known as A, B and C, who had taken their detailed and painful personal pregnancy experiences to the European Court of Human Rights, alleging that there were no relevant and appropriate services for them in Ireland.

An earlier landmark decision of the Supreme Court in 1992, in the case that became known as the 'X case', established the constitutional right to abortion if a pregnant woman's life was at risk, including through suicide, because of her pregnancy. Over a quarter of a century later, no government had introduced legislation to give effect to that ruling.

The European Court of Human Rights ruled that the State had infringed the rights of these women by not providing clear information on whether each of them was entitled to an abortion. Compensation was paid to each of them. The European Court of Human Rights gave the State an opportunity to respond offi-cially. The government decided in late December 2011 to appoint an expert group to advise on how to implement the judgment. That group, chaired by Mr Justice Sean Ryan, was mostly made up of doctors and lawyers, and I was appointed as a member.

As CMO, I had policy responsibility for bioethics, which is concerned with ethics in relation to healthcare and medical practice. This responsibility also included policy on human reproduction. My division therefore included a Bioethics Unit comprising the team of people who worked on these issues. On the issue of legislation for termination of pregnancy, we were ready in administrative terms, having the necessary preparatory work done to respond when the issue gained political focus, as it did periodically. We were hoping that a change in government policy or a change in the zeitgeist in relation to reproductive rights for women would bring an opportunity to make an advance.

On 28 October 2012, Savita Halappanavar died from sepsis, after her request for an abortion was denied by health-care staff who cited legal concerns. Her tragic and untimely death created a new context for public and political consideration of termination of pregnancy, and the right of a woman to make choices about her own health. The public outcry that resulted greatly influenced the government's thinking and brought a sense of urgency to the issue.

Among the options set out in the Ryan Report, which was published in December 2012, was legislation and regulations to enable termination of pregnancy to be provided in limited circumstances within the constraints of Article 40.3.3 of the Constitution. This is what ultimately became the Protection of Life in Pregnancy Act of 2013.

The provisions for access to abortion services in that 2013 Act were narrow. There were three in total: one for risk to life on the grounds of physical health; one for risk to life on the grounds of mental health (the risk of suicide); and one relating to emergency situations. These were the grounds on which termination would be legally permissible, and each of those specific grounds was prescriptive about the process that would be put into train. Abortion services outside these circumstances would continue to be illegal.

This was the first time abortion had been provided for in law in Ireland. Having a law on the statute books was a significant moment. However, the grounds for termination were so narrow that, in reality, few women could possibly benefit from access to termination of pregnancy. As a result, women continued to travel outside the State in significant numbers for terminations and continued to put their lives at risk.

* * *

One important principle of the 2013 Act was that it recognised that a medical practitioner could form a 'reasonable opinion' (defined in the Act as being an opinion formed in good faith which has regard to the need to preserve unborn human life as far as practicable). There was pressure and debate behind the scenes and in public to set out specific criteria and conditions for an opinion – for example relating to diseases, risks, conditions, etc. But none of that is reflected in the Act. Instead, the Act invested trust in the reasonable opinion formed in good faith of an attending medical practitioner of an appropriate specialism.

That was and still is crucial. I saw it as my duty as CMO to protect the principles of reasonable opinion and good faith as critical elements of medical practice in general, not just in relation to women's health. Unlike many other regulated health professions, the law in Ireland has not tried to set out a scope of practice that specifies how doctors should practise medicine. Rather, the Medical Council, with which a doctor must register, sets out guidance on professional standards and ethics. I believe that is a good thing. These principles were reflected in the 2013 Act and later carried forward to the 2018 legislation.

Ultimately, the 2013 Act provided for up to three doctors to confer and agree on grounds for access to termination. However, at one point during the development of the legislation, I can recall a political case – clearly coming from a perspective of resistance – being made to have three doctors agree on a decision, and for that decision to then be confirmed by a separate panel of three more doctors. Any woman who wished to appeal a decision would have to begin the process again, with three new doctors. That meant potentially up to 12 doctors being involved before a decision for a single woman who – as defined in the language of that Act – was someone facing 'real and substantial risk of loss of her life'. That might be hard to believe now, given how far we have come, but it shows the perspectives that existed at the time.

Another key feature of the 2013 Act is the limited information that is required to be submitted to the Minister for Health in respect of each termination. There were those who called for extensive information to be reported to the minister on each case, including the woman's Personal Public Service number (PPSN). I believed these demands were not in the interest of the women who might require the services the legislation was seeking to introduce. While it was up to the legislature to decide on the detail of the bill that led to the Act, we were in a position to influence it. We tried and failed to make a case that notification in relation to individual cases was not necessary. The next best outcome, therefore, was to do what we could to ensure that such information was kept to a minimum. The information required by the final Act in a notification ended up being quite limited. It comprised four elements: the section of the Act under which the termination would take place (i.e. the grounds); the date; the Medical Council number of the certifying practitioners; and the woman's county of residence.

That notification requirement was also reflected in the subsequent 2018 Act. This means that the annual report of notifications which the Minister of Health is required to lay before the houses of the Oireachtas each year is very short. We were pleased that we had managed to keep these provisions in the Act very minimal so as to protect the confidentiality of women and their doctors. In the first few years, those annual reports confirmed that somewhere between 20 and 30 terminations took place annually under the 2013 Act.

The principle of abortion in defined circumstances had been established. The 2013 Act did not deal with the public health and patient safety issue of lack of access to appropriate services that I described earlier – that would need a broadening of grounds of access to termination of pregnancy. But that in turn required the Constitution to change.

* * *

In November 2014, a 26-year-old woman, Natasha Perie, was pronounced dead, and then kept on life support for almost another four weeks, because she was 15 weeks pregnant. The doctors in her case were concerned about the implications of the Eighth Amendment and if it might prevent them from switching off her life support.

It was a shocking case. Natasha was dead but she was effect-ively being treated as a living incubator. When we heard about the case, I remember a meeting with the HSE where we expressed concern in the strongest terms about what was happening. Ultimately the family had to bring their case to a court to seek a decision to allow Natasha's life support to be switched off. Although an unusual case, it showed the impact of the prevailing constitutional position on medical practice. Natasha Perie's case also had a considerable effect on public and government thinking.

* * *

In 2016, the government established a Citizens' Assembly to consider and advise on a possible referendum on Article 40.3.3. There were 99 citizen members of the assembly, which was chaired by Ms Justice Mary Laffoy. These members were chosen at random from the electoral register to represent the views of the people of Ireland, and were broadly representative of society as reflected in the most recent census, including age, gender, social class, regional spread, etc.

Looking back, it seems clear that this set in motion a chain of events that was always going to lead to the services we now have in place. However, it felt anything but inevitable at the time. The assembly members spent five weekends considering the issues and duly produced a report with recommendations to remove and replace Article 40.3.3 with a provision that enabled legislation on termination of pregnancy to be introduced.

That recommendation from the Assembly was then referred to a specially convened Joint Oireachtas Committee on the Eighth Amendment of the Constitution to consider it. The Joint Oireachtas Committee in turn produced its recommendations. A final report from a Committee of politicians related to termination of pregnancy was no certainty – but it happened. It may have recommended something that was narrower than the recommendations of the Citizens' Assembly, but it was a final report and it was grounds for progress to be made.

That report was published on 23 December 2017. I knew that the political intention would be to have a referendum take place prior to the summer of 2018 to allow time for the law to be passed and services to be commenced at the start of 2019. This would require a great deal of work in a short time frame, but we were prepared.

At the start of January 2018, we drew up a detailed timetable and work plan that encompassed the referendum, any necessary legislation and the possible development of new services such that they could commence on 1 January 2019. We set out the timetable in a memorandum for government to be tabled by the minister at the first cabinet meeting of 2018. We subsequently provided updated memoranda for the minister to apprise the government on the progress of work in accordance with the timetable at almost every cabinet meeting in the first half of 2018.

We knew that if Article 40.3.3 was not repealed at this opportunity, it might be years before we could get back to that point again. We, as the responsible officials, could not become the reason the service would be delayed. Whatever about the implications for us, the important reality would be thousands of women denied a service for years to come. We knew we could not drop the ball. We had every bit of determination necessary to deliver on this.

One critical part of the plan was that the policy paper setting out the government's detailed intended wording of the bill providing for expanded access to termination of pregnancy would be published in advance of the referendum so that the people could see and understand what the government intended the Oireachtas to legislate for, before the referendum was held. As a result, it would be clear to everyone what changes were intended by government if the referendum was passed.

When the country voted on 25 May 2018, two-thirds of voters chose to repeal Article 40.3.3. That was a wonderful moment. I was in my local having a pint with my dad when the result was confirmed. Clodagh, who was 17 at the time, was very engaged by the whole issue. I remember her complaining that she felt so strongly about it and it mattered so much to young girls and women and yet she couldn't vote. She and her friends bought 'Repeal' jumpers and went to Dublin Castle to celebrate and to feel a part of the change. Somehow, they managed to end up right at the front of the crowd almost beside Leo Varadkar in the press photos and television news.

The team in my division took great pride in having played a central part, albeit invisibly, in keeping the process on track. But we also knew that we had to push on with the detailed plans for services to begin on 1 January 2019.

While the government's intention for the bill had been published in the form of a policy paper which was published in advance of the referendum, the actual bill took almost all the remainder of 2018 to finalise and to be enacted by the Oireachtas. It was a very sensitive bill that had to clarify and define many things, for example the definition of '12 weeks', so that the bill that was enacted could be implemented in practice. A plan also needed to be developed to put the services in place: guidelines were required; a contract for service with GPs had to be developed and negotiated; and hospital pathways of care had to be developed. Medicines had to be licensed for use. Training had to be put in place to provide for a service which would take place in hospitals, general practices and clinics in the community. This was the work of the second half of 2018.

The service commenced, as planned, on 1 January 2019. More than six and a half thousand women up and down the country used those services in 2019. Ireland now had a modern, safe, primarily community-based, early pregnancy termination of pregnancy service for thousands of women. Naturally, as a father of a young woman I see this in personal terms. Clodagh and her generation of young women will never have to suffer the indignities of the women before them who faced a very difficult and risky journey overseas for a vital health service at an already difficult time in their lives.

There is still work to be done. Only one in six GPs provide this service. We still have counties in which there is no service. Many hospitals have yet to commence the service, and even in those that do, it is via a small number of practitioners. In part, I think the penalties and the overly fastidious procedural requirements of the Act may be off-putting for many doctors.

The legislation was the subject of a review which was published in April 2023. I hope this will allow those provisions that act as inhibitors to involvement of doctors can be revisited. I would also hope that in that review the requirement of a three-day wait can be removed. It patronisingly suggests that a woman seeking a termination of pregnancy needs to 'go off and have a good think for herself'. It serves no medical purpose whatsoever.

I feel strongly that there is no room for complacency. We know by now, looking at other countries, that progress in this area can be lost as well as gained. We need to expand the numbers providing these services, and copper-fasten and consolidate the hard-won progress that these changes represent.

* * *

When I look back, although my role on this occasion was not publicly visible, I feel privileged and proud of the enormous work we did together. Privileged because, as a doctor, I had a unique and direct role that very few doctors ever do to shape a ground-breaking law relating to medical practice. Pride, because as a doctor I was centrally involved over many years on advancing women's health policy and legislation and access to reproductive health services which culminated in the implementation of a modern, safe, largely primary care-based service that women can access in their own community and at early stages in pregnancy. It is one good example of why I did the job that I did and why I loved it so much.

It may be a cliché, but this really was a team effort. Much of the path was laid by a relatively small unit in my division of the Department of Health called the Bioethics Unit. This was a dedicated and experienced team led by principal officer Geraldine Luddy, who had been director of the Women's Health Council, which was subsumed into the Department of Health in the wake of the economic downturn.

Geraldine is one of the best colleagues I ever had the privilege of working with. She was passionate, committed, capable and great fun to work with. Ronan Horgan, a genial Corkonian, was the legal adviser in the Department of Health assigned to work with us on this. We three and the staff of the Bioethics Unit worked extremely closely throughout the period leading to the establishment of the new service in January 2019.

The team was very well supported by a great group of committed legal brains in the Attorney General's office. My insight into and understanding of their role and my appreciation of their professionalism and expertise grew enormously over those intense months. They included Jennifer Payne, Christine O'Rourke and Margaret Kelleher. There was a great *esprit de corps* between us all and we had many very long but enjoyable meetings. I recall in particular one all-day meeting over the Easter weekend, when the country was snowbound, when we slid into Merrion Street and sat in the cold basement, with no coffee, going through an early draft of the bill line by line.

This was a very pressurised and intense programme of work, and the work just before the referendum was particularly so. The timetable was very tight, and the team worked almost every weekend in the first half of 2018. We had many conference calls with one another to discuss the policy and the bill we were working on. Zoom wasn't yet a feature of our lives. I remember Ronan Horgan describing the scene in his back garden – his children were building a snowman and he wanted to join them, but we were too busy.

We had highly confidential discussions with medical experts in all the relevant fields. We never identified the people we went to for advice, but we relied heavily on them and their willingness to take calls, attend meetings and read material with very little notice. I pay tribute to them and their altruism.

There was a significant reliance on a small group of people in the HSE, particularly after the referendum, when attention turned to developing the services to be made legal by the legislation. This included in particular Dr Peter McKenna, Director of the Women and Infants Health Programme, as well as Pat Healy and his small team. These people did heroic work. Committed public servants doing everything they could to make a service available to the public.

CHAPTER FIFTEEN

Difficult Times

2017–2021

THE SECOND FOUR YEARS of Emer's illness moved at a different pace from the first four years. She experienced a much greater degree of pain almost continually. New lesions formed in different places more frequently. Each time she ran into difficulty in a specific location because of a new lesion, her treatment would be adapted to deal with what that difficulty demanded. It might be pain relief or radiotherapy. Some of these lesions were in places where their effect was temporarily disabling. Sometimes, therefore, she might need support for walking, or use of mobility aids like a wheelchair.

On Good Friday 2017, she developed very severe back pain and shooting sciatica-like pain down one side that she described as being like electric shocks. The real concern this immediately gave rise to was spinal cord compression, something that constitutes a medical emergency because it can lead to paralysis if the compression continues or gets worse.

I phoned the myeloma nurse in St James's Hospital, Emma Hayes, who, like all the myeloma specialist nurses we dealt with over the years, was wonderful. She was our first point of contact. She advised Emer to come in and told me that she would set about arranging an emergency CT. Emer couldn't walk properly, and making our way down the corridor to the X-ray department was extremely difficult and painful.

The first news was very worrying. At one point on that first afternoon there were a number of consultants in the room – not just haematology but radiology, neurology and radiation oncology – all looking at the scan of Emer's spine and all very concerned, as we were. Fortunately, the clinical examination was more reassuring than the scans had been. It turned out to be not quite full spinal cord compression. Emer was given radiotherapy and high-dose steroids through the weekend, and some of the pain and the worrying 'electric shock' sensations settled down over the course of a week or ten days.

One positive thing about myeloma is that it is very radio-sensitive, meaning the lesions respond very well to radiotherapy. Multiple myeloma means there are multiple other myelomas, and it isn't therefore feasible to give radiation as systemic treatment to the whole body or bone marrow system; systemic treatment depends on chemotherapy. Radiotherapy is used in specific lesions when they cause, or are likely to cause, local effects.

Once the pain had stabilised to some extent, Emer was admitted to Our Lady's Hospice in Harold's Cross for the first time. The purpose was as a respite admission; to take time to recover under the direction of Norma O'Leary and her team and their expertise in the control of pain.

That, in my recollection, was the heralding of that second four years. During the first half of her time with the illness, the pace of new lesions was slower, and pain control was much better. In the second half, lesions came more rapidly, and pain was an ever more challenging issue.

* * *

That first admission to the hospice was very hard for all of us.

That is no reflection on the hospice itself. The rooms are large, comfortable and private. Each has a patio door that leads to a lovely courtyard with an outdoor table and chairs to allow people to experience the serenity of the beautifully kept gardens. One and all, the nurses, doctors, carers, catering staff, volunteers, counsellors, physiotherapists and occupational therapists are wonderful people. So caring and considerate. Always with a kind word and a smile. All the patients would undoubtedly rather be somewhere else, but when you are there and need to be, it really does feel like a very special place.

Emer and I both understood – and we explained to Clodagh and Ronan – what palliative care is. We knew that it isn't always end-of-life care. It plays an important role in providing respite for people who need expertise in symptom control and the input of a wider team of professionals, including physiotherapists, occupational therapists, social work counsellors, nurses and others. And yet, despite all the knowledge and understanding we had, that feeling that we were entering into a new phase, crossing a threshold, was still there.

That was much in my mind, and I know it was in Emer's too. But I didn't want to bring it to the fore at that precise moment. We had to first of all get over the day of admission and its symbolic significance. In talking to Emer, I tried to be very matter of fact: 'This is just something we need to do, another service we need to avail of, to get you back on your feet.'

At this time, Emer was 49. Her fiftieth birthday was coming up – 31 May 2017. Martha had turned 50 on 3 April, but Emer hadn't been able to get to the celebrations. So Martha and our close friends Eleanor and Barbara took the party to Emer in the hospice. They brought a beautifully decorated cake with an edible stethoscope on top.

That was the first time Martha had seen Emer since she was admitted to St James's Hospital on Good Friday, 14 April. I remember standing in my kitchen talking to Martha after that visit, and her saying to me how worried she was about Emer; that she didn't think she was going to see her fiftieth birthday. That was only weeks away.

That is how bad things were then. Emer was so unwell. There was a strong sense that her disease was progressing quickly. She was on a great deal of medication along with the radiotherapy, and there were increasingly debilitating side effects, particularly from dexamethasone, a very strong steroid.

Somehow, Emer rallied, and by her fiftieth at the end of May, she was out of the hospice and home. Happily, she made a habit of defying predictions. That summer, I took as long a break as I could in July and August, and we got to Ballybunion, which was always a joy for Emer. Looking back, those were good months. After Kerry, Emer spent a lot of time that summer in the garden, and with the children. There was still a sense – just as there had been after the trip to Boston – of options and possibilities within her treatment. That changed over the winter and into the next few years.

More often, new lesions would crop up and would escape the control of the systemic treatment, the chemotherapy. These would produce specific symptoms and have to be dealt with individually, usually by radiotherapy. The blend of drugs began to change increasingly frequently over this time, as they stopped working or the side effects became too much, and there was a new sense that we were running out of options.

At one point Emer developed a lump on her head that grew very quickly. When examined clinically it was clear it was in the bone of the skull and expanding outwards from there. The skull contains marrow and is therefore a common site for myeloma lesions. A scan showed it was extending inwards to an even greater extent, to the point where it was pressing on her brain. She had no choice but to have radiotherapy, which might cause her to lose her hair for the second time. The psychic pain Emer suffered over the loss of her hair was very hard for her to bear. Unfortunately, there was no option but to go ahead with the radiotherapy. Happily, she had a very good response to it, and that lesion practically disappeared, and very quickly. Efforts were made to minimise hair loss but, alas, they weren't successful.

Later, much closer to the end of her life, when questions around radiotherapy to her head arose again, the thought of losing her hair once more was part of her decision to refuse it.

* * *

In the summer of 2018, there was further recurrence of pain in Emer's back. Colin Doherty was away, as it happened, and in his absence another neurologist was involved in her care; Siobhan Hutchinson, who was also a good friend from UCD and St Vincent's. She was wonderful. A serious question arose again about the stability of Emer's spine, and the possibility of surgery to stabilise it was mooted. That would have meant admission to Beaumont. We had her bag packed, ready to go. We understood that there could be no guarantee of success, and that the surgery could perhaps make a bad situation even worse. In the end, the surgeon said he wasn't prepared to operate, on the basis that 'If I go in, I don't see how I can come back out . . .' Some of my surgical friends say the mark of a good surgeon is knowing when not to operate. We felt the benefit of that expertise on that occasion. We went with more radiotherapy instead, and her spinal symptoms settled for a time.

Emer's vertebrae were being effectively destroyed one by one by this unrelenting disease. They were collapsing and re-healing and collapsing again. And Emer was losing height as the vertebrae in her back collapsed. When I met her first, she was tall – five foot eleven – and so striking looking. I would say she was five foot five or six when she died. She lost that height, just as she lost everything else.

Bit by bit, over the course of those eight years, myeloma robbed her of everything. Of life, obviously, and time, but also of how she looked; how she felt about herself; her energy and vitality. It was the thief of everything she held dear.

* * *

We were now into a back-and-forth between home, hospital and hospice. Something would happen that meant Emer would need to go into hospital, and from there she would go to the hospice. There were many bad days. Days when she felt absolutely awful or was in unbearable pain. Days when we got bad news in hospital – for example, her paraprotein levels would have gone up unexpectedly, and that, we knew, signified further progression of the disease.

How we responded as a family was how Emer responded. She had an incredible ability to keep going. On the day she received bad news or disappointing results, she could be very upset, but then she had an extraordinary capacity to push it all to one side and get on with what she wanted to do. She would talk it out with me – often in the hospital or on the journey home – and then was able to compartmentalise and focus on being with the kids and being available for them.

She was like that right up to the very end. Even when she couldn't walk or move much, when she was only able to be in a chair or a bed, she was there for them, to talk and listen. They would sit on the edge of the bed and chat to her. If she was waking them in the morning – and it was such an important thing for her, to be physically able to get into their bedrooms – she would sit on the edge of their beds and chat to them before they got up.

And that was normal family life for most of the time. Whatever Emer was able to do, she did. On days when she needed to rest more and move less, she did that and we went to her. We were always open when talking to Clodagh and Ronan about how she was getting on, what the doctors were saying, and what that meant. This was all just part of the regular conversations we had. We talked about it as much or as little as seemed relevant on any given day. It was folded into the fabric of our lives, and those lives continued around it.

After all, with something like myeloma, you're managing a slowly evolving situation. With this kind of cancer, Emer was effectively tethered to the hospital, going from month to month; that is unlike some cancers, where initial treatment can lead to cure or very long periods of remission when people regain much of their functionality and their lives.

We adapted as everyone adapts to their circumstances. You just do whatever it is you can do at any given moment.

*　*　*

Clodagh's Leaving Certificate, in 2019, was the last pre-Covid Leaving Certificate. Approaching Clodagh's exams, it was obvious to me that Emer was getting worse. She couldn't manage as much as she had been. She had been in the hospice in the spring of that year, and was still quite symptomatic, and limited in what she could do.

I had to take time off work in June, to be there during the exam period. Ronan was in the Gaeltacht in Connemara for three weeks, so it was just the three of us. I made the journey alone to visit him on the two Sundays he was away as Emer wasn't well enough.

Until this point, it had felt as though new lesions were arising every six months or so. From then on, these intervals began to get shorter and shorter. The lesions came more often, and there was much less recovery in between. Emer could no longer get back to where she had been before something new would crop up.

At some point towards the end of 2019, she got a lesion at the top of her right arm that was very debilitating. She lost the use of her shoulder and arm. Radiotherapy helped with the pain, but the disability largely remained. She wasn't able to drive very much after that, and couldn't do the things she wanted to around the house or for the kids. By now we had a lot of devices in the house – power-assisted chairs, grab rails and so on. Home visits from the occupational therapist and physiotherapist really helped to give us equipment and also techniques that made it easier – but not easy – for Emer to manage day-to-day living and to be at home.

Emer never got back to functional independence, which was deeply, painfully frustrating for her. And if I am honest – as I feel it is important to be – it was difficult for me too. I do not mean in any way to compare what I went through with what Emer was going through. There is obviously no possible comparison. And my first thoughts, always, in this are with Emer and what she suffered. But I believe it is important to acknowledge that a slow demise of a loved one over a long period of time brings challenges to everyone in a family. It was a wonderful thing that Emer was able to see Ronan grow to the age of 18; to see him into his Leaving Certificate year; to watch Clodagh start college – but it also placed great pressure on us as a family for many years.

There were times when I felt that I didn't know how much longer I could keep doing what I was doing. I could feel the strain of managing both work and home. At times it felt like I wasn't doing either well enough. But then I would remind myself that everyone facing these circumstances has these moments of doubt and low confidence. I would take my inspiration from Emer and pick myself up and keep going.

I find even writing that now very difficult. It feels disloyal. It feels as though this takes away from my gratitude that Emer remained with us as long as she did. The reality is that the effect of something as debilitating as myeloma, or any serious chronic illness, changes the nature of your relationship. A relationship – a marriage – that has been equal becomes unequal, divided into a person who needs care and a person who is caring. That is how it evolved for Emer and me. And I know we both struggled with that. That was not where we had started, that is not how we ever were together.

It is hard to be the person who is cared for. There is so much of yourself – your sense of pride, self-confidence, independence and dignity – that you have to put aside. When that care is provided by your spouse or partner it can be very hard on both of you. I'm not saying the challenges are equal or comparable. But they are real.

One of the things I learned through this is that an illness like Emer's impacts the whole family, affecting different people in different ways. I think of the enormous number of carers and families under daily strain who don't have the support that I was lucky enough to have – whether those supports are friends and family, workplace or my knowledge of how the system works.

From Emer's point of view, the indignity involved in submitting to being cared for by someone you love, with whom you've had an intimate relationship, is an enormous shift. She had no choice but to allow this, but that doesn't mean she was resigned to it. Being in need of such help was deeply undermining to her sense of independence. Naturally she wanted to hold on to every little shred of that. There were periods when she couldn't do very much for herself. And as the years went on there were more and more of those times. She wasn't able to provide for herself, prepare food or dress herself. The impact that had on her, on her sense of self-worth, and the way she was with the children, was very difficult.

I didn't always cope with it as well as I would have liked. There were times I got frustrated or annoyed. I might have wanted something to be done in a particular way because it made it easier or faster for me, and Emer might have a different view. We weren't always pulling in the same direction.

The truth is, it is easier for the carer if the person being cared for fully submits to their way of doing things. Emer didn't. She had her own views on how things should be done – even small matters, like where she wanted to sit, how to store her medications in her medication bag, or when she wanted to have her dinner – and she wasn't prepared to simply give these up. Little tensions arose, moments of dispute. Sometimes I felt annoyed that she didn't recognise that it might have been easier for me to do it in my way. But what I was failing to recognise was that that would be taking away even more of her independence.

I'm not proud of that. In fact, it is very hard to think about it now. To remember and understand how difficult things were in the moment, that I could have become so frustrated. But I think it is important to be honest about it. Emer and I always made sure we got around to discussing and reviewing those things. We talked them out and would agree on how better to manage the challenges. But we didn't always manage to prevent them.

Mentally, I was in two places – work and home – and unable to fully switch off from either. Once the pandemic began, Emer spent a lot of time reading media reports about Covid, and following social media. She did this because she was terrified. She was particularly vulnerable to Covid. The nature of her disease placed her at the very top of the list of those at risk. She had a sense of dread. She had survived for so long with her disease by then; she had fought every step to get as much time as possible with the children; and now this virus, which had appeared out of the blue, was a real and very substantial threat to her.

That was immensely difficult for her. And occasionally for me. I would come home from work, having talked and thought about Covid all day, and I would want nothing more than to forget about it. But Emer would be keen to hear everything about what I was hearing and seeing. She wanted, as a public health doctor, to get as good an understanding of the risk of the disease and any possible news on vaccination developments. That is all extremely understandable.

* * *

Life shrank ever further in these months and years. I had given up GAA coaching in about 2016 as I just wasn't able to commit to doing that on top of everything else. Now I began to scale back anything that was left.

Emer was able to see Clodagh out of school and into university, which was a huge thing for her. She didn't get that far with Ronan. The one consolation is that, by the time he started his Leaving Certificate year, it was clear to both of us that he was doing well and was a good student. Academic achievement was one thing we didn't have to worry about with Clodagh and Ronan. Ronan achieved great results in spite of Emer's death in February of his Leaving Certificate year. He is now studying actuarial and financial studies in UCD. Emer would have been so proud.

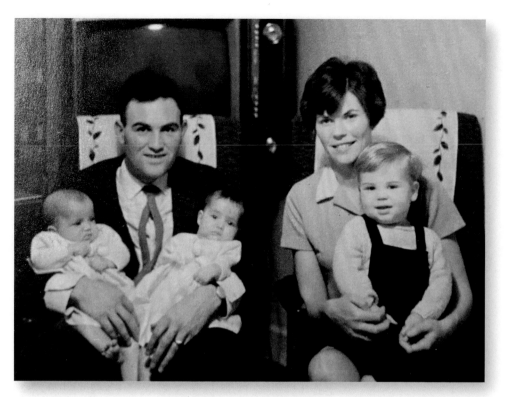

At home in Baldoyle, Dublin, in the summer of 1969. Mum and Dad with their Irish triplets!

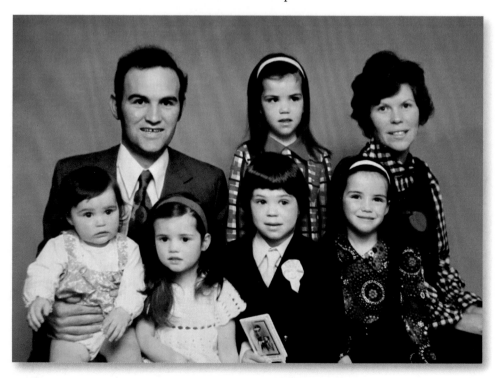

My First Communion, Castletroy, Limerick, 1974.

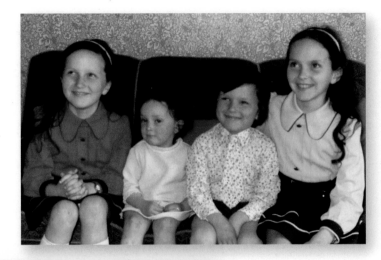

Emer, on the left, with siblings Niamh, Ronan and Orla.

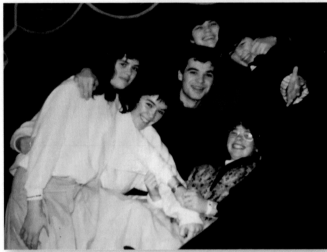

My sisters and I having a laugh at home, circa 1985.

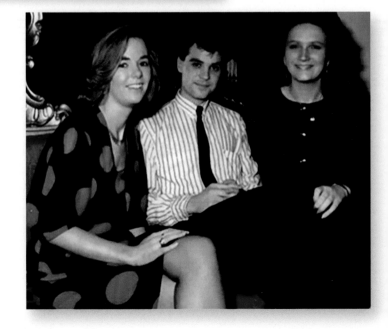

Martha, me and Emer, circa 1989.

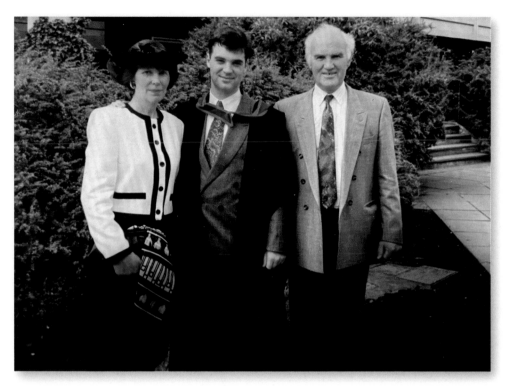

With my parents Brigid and Liam on my graduation day, UCD, June 1991.

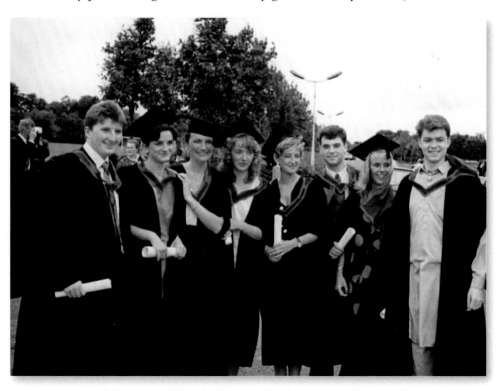

Graduation Day, UCD, June 1991. From left: Mark Rowe, Eleanor, Emer, Emer Henry, Barbara, me, Martha and Colin.

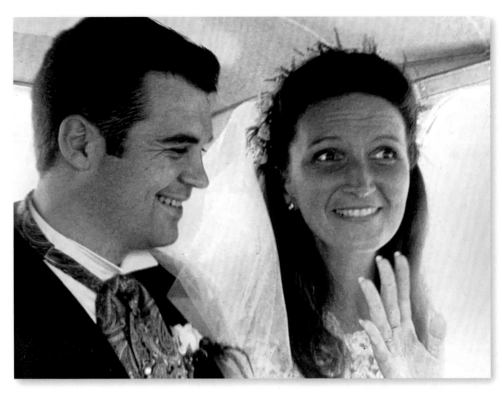

On our wedding day, 19 August 1995.

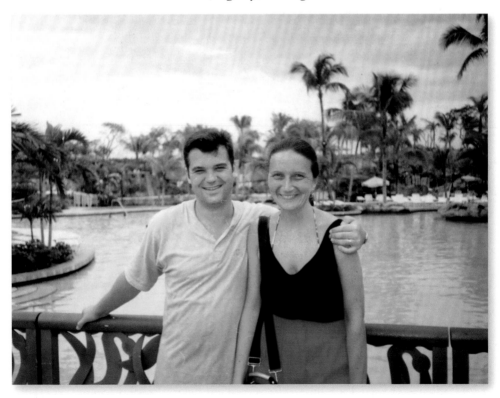

On honeymoon in Paradise Island, Bahamas, August 1995.

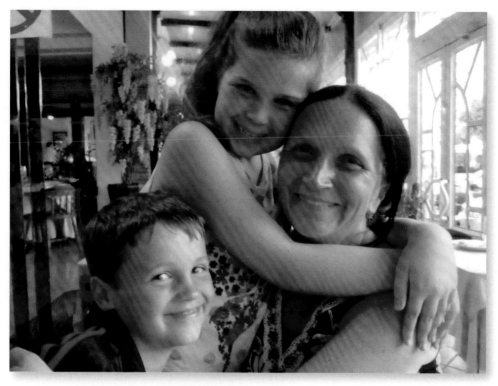

Emer with Clodagh and
Ronan, Benalmadena,
Easter 2008.

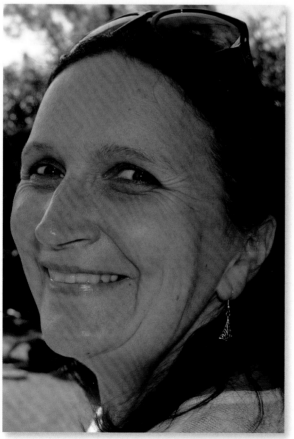

Emer, May 2012.

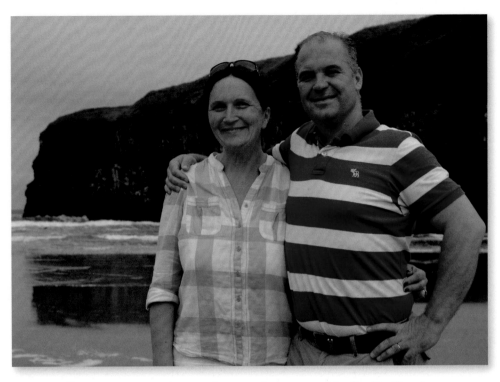

Emer, wearing a shirt we later made into a teddy. Ladies Beach, Ballybunion, 2012.

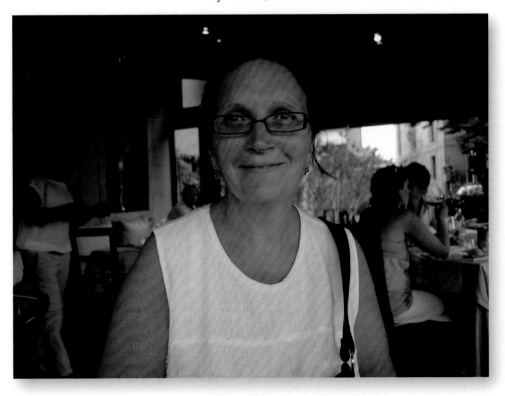

Emer one month before diagnosis in August 2012, at Lake Garda in Italy.

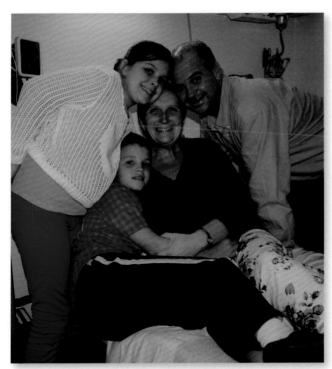

Ronan's 10th birthday,
St James's Hospital,
19 September 2012.

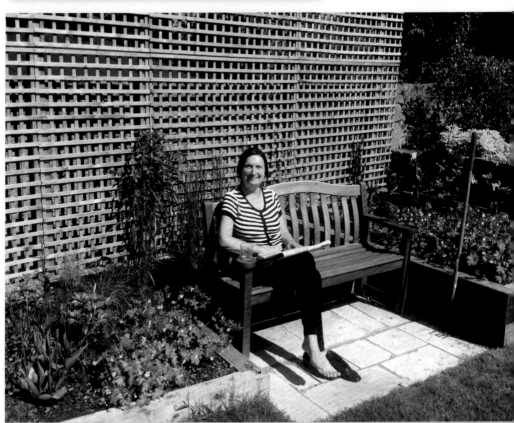

Emer relaxing in the garden in early summer 2013.

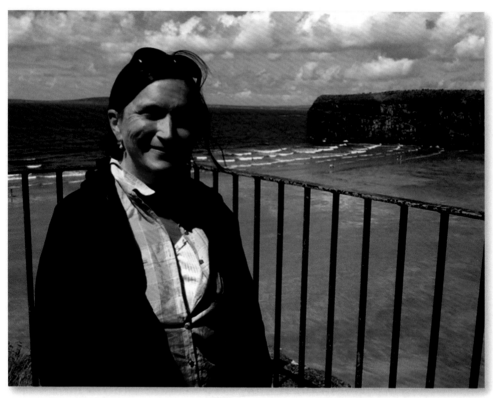

Emer at Ballybunion Ladies Beach in July 2013.

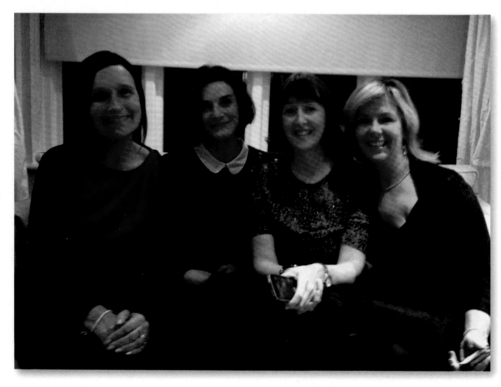

Emer with our great friends Eleanor, Barbara and Martha.

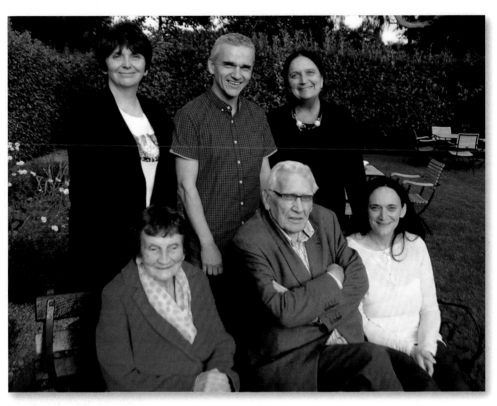

The Feely family: (from left) Orla, Ita, Ronan, Frank, Emer and Niamh, October 2016.

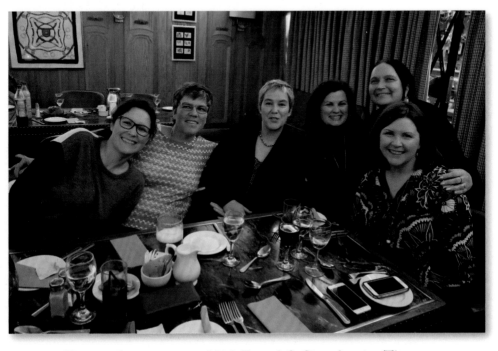

Emer with my sisters in 2016. From left: Sinead, twins Therese and Aileen, Breda, Emer and Aoife.

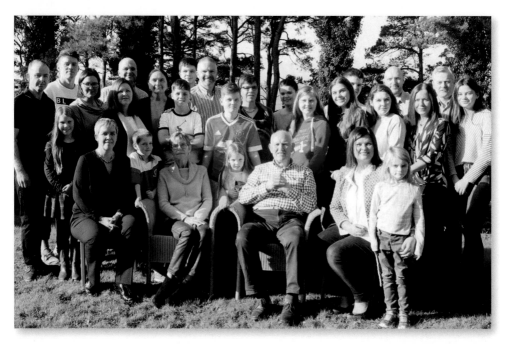

The Holohan family gathering, Terryglass, Co. Tipperary, October 2016.

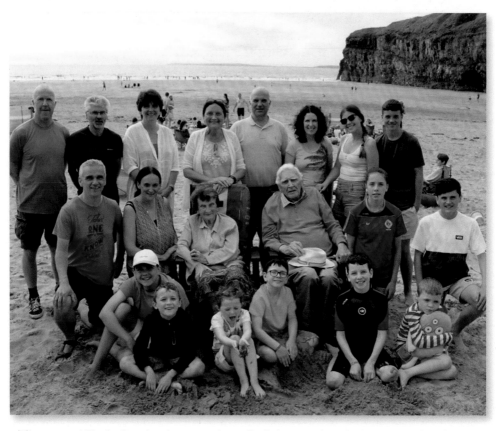

The annual Feely family photograph on Ballybunion beach in 2018, taken by my friend Dr Tadhg Crowley of Kilkenny...and Kerry!

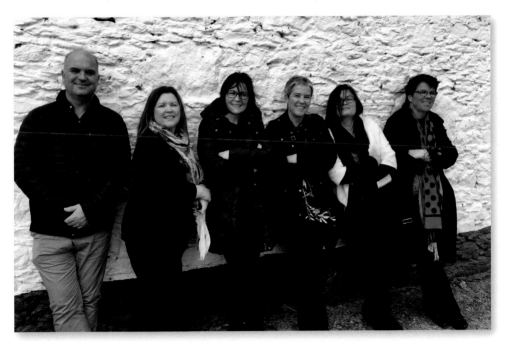

Together in my mother's home place in Cappamore in 2017 with Aoife, Sinead, Aileen, Breda and Therese.

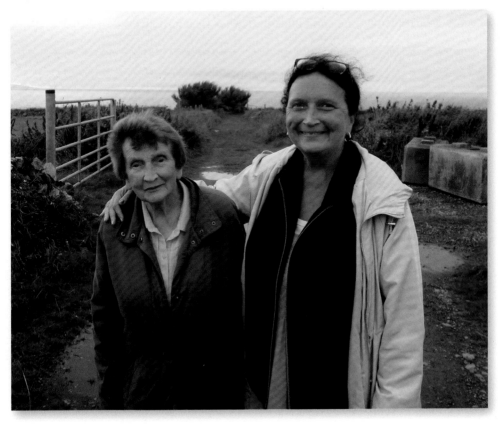

Emer and her mother Ita, Ballybunion, 2018.

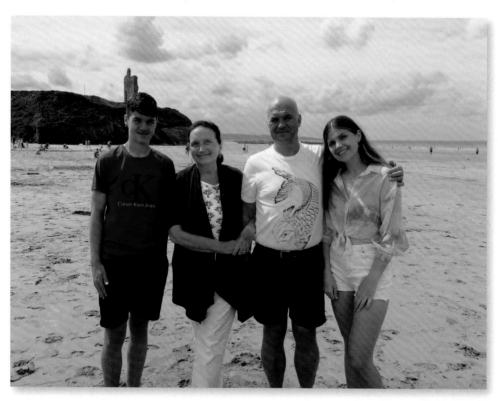

Ronan, Emer, me and Clodagh, Ladies Beach, Ballybunion, 2019.

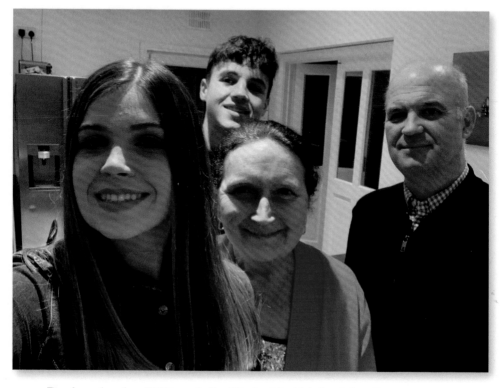

Ready to head to Dillinger's for Clodagh's 19th birthday, January 2020.

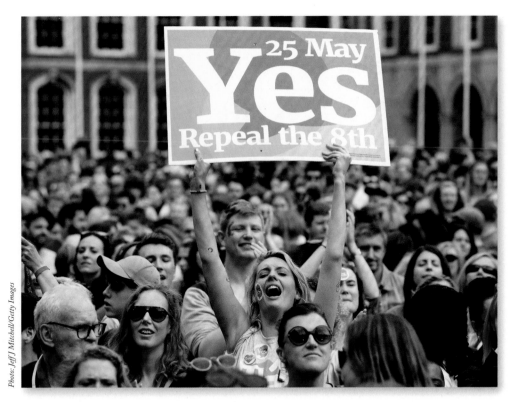

Crowds celebrate the result of the Eighth Amendment Referendum at at Dublin Castle.

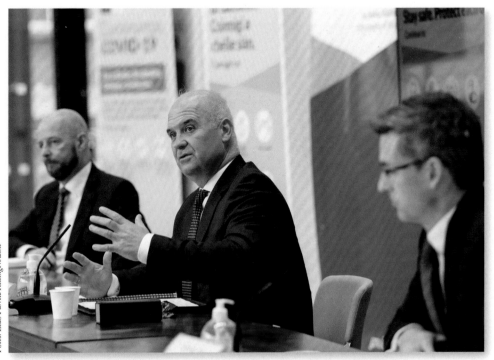

Prof Philip Nolan, me and Dr Ronan Glynn at a Covid-19 press conference.

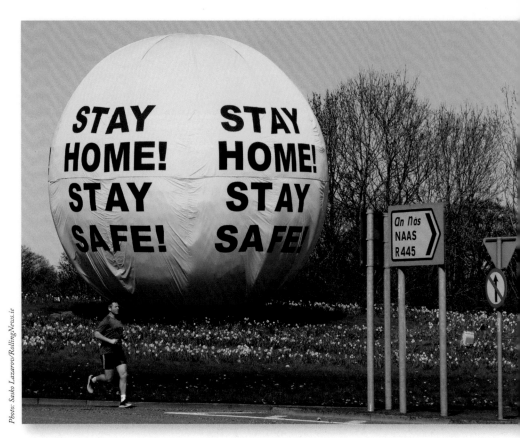

Photo: Sasko Lazarov/RollingNews.ie

The Covid-19 yellow was everywhere in Ireland thanks to Deirdre Watters.

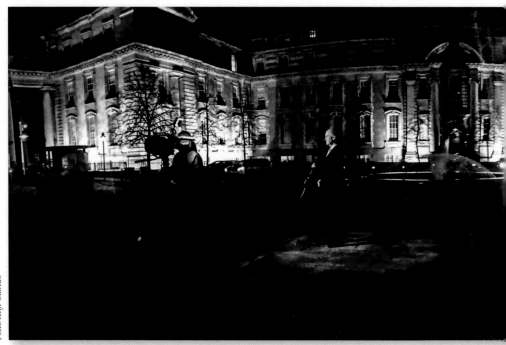

Photo: Aoife Gillivan

Live on the Nine O'Clock News, 29 March 2020.

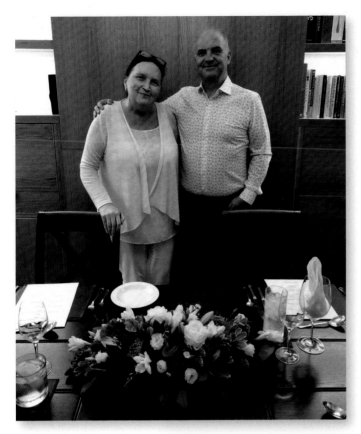

Our 25th and last wedding anniversary, 19 August 2020.

A tribute to Emer on Ballybunion Ladies beach, 19 February 2021, thanks to Greg and Una Ryan and the people of Ballybunion.

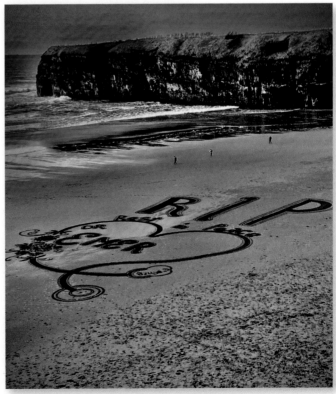

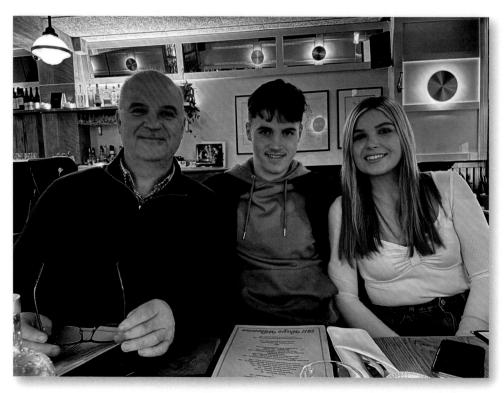

With Clodagh and Ronan for Clodagh's 22nd Birthday, 10 January 2023, Dillinger's restaurant, Ranelagh.

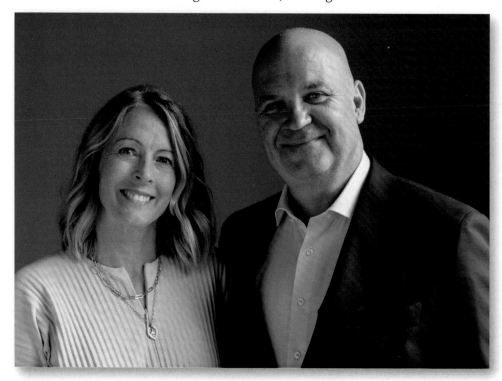

Ciara and me, summer 2023.

I know he is there, and Clodagh is in physiotherapy in Trinity College Dublin, because of all the love, support and encouragement from Emer throughout their lives and their school years.

* * *

In June 2020 Emer went back into the hospice. She was discharged on Saturday 11 July. Over the remainder of that summer she improved somewhat. We didn't get to Ballybunion, she wasn't well enough to travel that far, but she spent time in the garden and was relatively okay, physically.

The day she came home from the hospice, Emer insisted she wanted to call to see her mother, Ita. Our journey home takes us past Emer's parents' house, where she grew up. I didn't want to stop. I wanted to get Emer home, and suggested that it would be better to get her settled and then invite her parents to call around in the evening, but Emer was insistent.

She hadn't seen her parents in a fortnight as they hadn't been able to visit the hospice, because of Covid. I've written previously about Emer's relationship with her mother. How close they were. How often they talked to one another. She was determined now to see her, even if it was only to call to the door and have Ita come out.

So we did as Emer wished, and Ita came out for a chat. It was a lovely summer's day. Ita stood at the car window chatting happily to Emer for ten minutes or so, going through all the grandchildren, Clodagh and Ronan and all the family updates.

Emer never saw her mother fit and well again. The following Wednesday, Ita had a profound stroke, out of the blue, having had no serious medical issues throughout her life. Ita was admitted to St James's Hospital and she spent a very long time there. While she was in the hospital, I could bring Emer to see her. Later, she was moved to a long-term care bed in Our

Lady's Hospice and Care Services in Harold's Cross. Ita never recovered. She regained some of her functions but had very limited awareness. Life changed completely for Frank. He was mentally fully fit although he had some medical issues to contend with. Ita had done everything for him, and now, at the age of 89, he had to learn how to cook and to live alone and this was just awful for him. It makes me think of how common a situation that is. Two elderly people living together independently but interdependently. All it takes is one event for one of them, in this case Ita's stroke, to bring it all to an abrupt end.

*　*　*

When I left work at the start of that summer of 2020, I had no sense of when I might return. I believed that Emer would not live for much longer. Yet three months later, I chose to go back to work. Emer had defied the odds again and was now the one pushing me to go back to work. For Emer, me being at home was not the natural order of things. It felt like confirmation for her that she was not well.

And so back I went. Three weeks later, Emer had to go back into the hospice. That was a fateful admission. It was the beginning of the end.

CHAPTER SIXTEEN
The Arrival of Covid

BY THE TIME THE European Centre for Disease Prevention and Control (ECDC) published a paper called 'Pneumonia cases possibly associated with a novel coronavirus in Wuhan, China' on 9 January 2020, Emer was well into the second four-year phase of her illness. There was much in that report to cause concern. And still so much to be known and discovered.

By this time, Emer was on morphine all the time to control her ever-present pain, and had mobility problems caused by the more frequently occurring lesions. She was much more limited in the physical tasks she could carry out. At times the pain became too much, even for someone who had become so used to living with pain. She had a number of respite admissions to Our Lady's Hospice in Harold's Cross. Clodagh, Ronan and I were managing the house and Emer's needs without having to have additional home care services in place. We also had great support nearby from both sides of the family.

And then, on top of everything that was happening at home, these reports began to trickle in. They were immediately concerning.

The truth is, Covid couldn't have come at a worse time for Emer, or for our family. There was a part of me that thought,

I don't need this. Just as Emer was getting sicker, I was becoming more tethered to the job. And yet I never thought of leaving. That was Emer's decision as much as it was mine.

We had a lot of conversations about this. It was important to Emer that I stay, because she knew it was important for me, and because she believed that I could play an important role in dealing with the issues. She told me I couldn't just step away at a time like this. Also, being at work was confirmation for Emer that she could keep going. She clung to her independence. Me being at home meant she wasn't doing well. And she worried about me having to be away from the job for periods of time due to her illness. She had enough to worry about without also worrying about me and my job.

If Covid had happened during my first year or two as CMO, I would have found it much more challenging. Looking back, I managed swine flu as best I could, but it wasn't the event that Covid was to become. I don't want to make it sound like, 'Oh, nobody could have done this job except me.' But I was in a position to make a contribution that I think others might have struggled to make. I had been CMO for 12 years. I had worked with many Ministers for Health, and on many difficult issues. Taking on this task would require experience and a lack of fear. And I was in a position where I had all the relevant experience and was not fearful of the difficulties that I thought an issue of this kind would throw up.

Knowing that Emer believed in me and in what I had to offer at this strange time was a pivotal part of what enabled me to do the job in those very difficult few years.

* * *

At first, there wasn't much information about this new virus. In those early weeks, the reports were simply along the lines of 'there is something interesting-or-concerning going on in Wuhan . . .' On the evening of Clodagh's nineteenth birthday dinner in Ranelagh – 10 January – that was about as much as we really knew. The small number of reports I had seen at that point very much located this problem as belonging to Wuhan and China. That was certainly how the media reported it for some time. But if all the early reports of transmissibility were borne out, I knew it was only a matter of time before this disease would come to Ireland.

The fact that it was a coronavirus was somewhat surprising. Based on the swine flu experience and on probability, the expectation was for a global pandemic featuring some form of influenza. The risk of that remains. Avian influenza, for example, is a very severe illness. If it mutates in such a way as to enable it to spread effectively from human to human, that is going to be a very significant public health challenge for humanity.

But this time, that is not what happened. Instead SARS CoV-2, as it was officially named by WHO, was a new virus. And those early reports were immediately alarming. Since it was completely new, humans would not have natural immunity – the world's population was 'naive' in that sense. We had no drugs to treat it, and we didn't have a vaccine. And as far as we could infer from the data on severity and transmissibility that was coming from China, it seemed to represent a much greater public health threat than seasonal influenza, which in most years causes a winter epidemic that often results in significant excess winter mortality.

The potential for this to become something serious within a matter of weeks was very clear. I knew that it was just a matter of time before we were going to be dealing with it here in Europe, and in Ireland. We were in the run-up to an election, but Simon Harris was still in place as Minister for Health. Each week we prepared 'memoranda for information', as they are called, to keep cabinet apprised. These were then tabled at cabinet by Minister Harris. We indicated in these memoranda that this new virus was something to be aware of and be informed about, that we were carefully monitoring its spread, liaising with the WHO and ECDC and looking in detail at our preparedness plans. I felt that was more than sufficient at that time. With an election under way, there was understandably no great interest in the wider political implications at this stage.

Around mid-January, I began to have informal discussions with a group of people about what we were seeing. They were: Dr Ronan Glynn, deputy CMO; Dr Cillian de Gascun, consultant virologist and National Director of the National Virus Reference Laboratory (NVRL) in UCD; Dr Kevin Kelleher, Assistant National Director for Health Protection in the HSE; and John Cuddihy, Director of the health protection Surveillance Centre. They all later formed part of the NPHET.

I can recall, with no disrespect to these men, missing Dr Darina O'Flanagan, who had retired a few years previously. She was a towering figure in public health surveillance and infectious disease control and had an international reputation. She was a great person to have on your team in any infectious disease incident, and I had depended on her greatly during swine flu. I resolved to ask her to come out of retirement if this developed in the way we all feared it might. Within a couple of weeks, I made that telephone call and she joined my team immediately until the time I left my post in July 2022.

Over that January, we gathered in the evenings after everyone's working day via teleconference calls on our phones. We discussed what we had each learned. Around this time the ECDC and the WHO were updating summary assessments and providing guidance to member states every day. We were fully tuned into these.

Another key thing from those days was my calls with Mike Ryan, who was in a key position in WHO headquarters in Geneva and one of the key architects of the global response. While his focus was, of necessity, on the challenges for the entire world, he is an Irish man and was always willing to take an evening phone call to chat things through. The WHO had access to the detail of what was happening in those early days in Wuhan; what the early research was saying in terms of viral loads, reproduction numbers, severity, underlying risks, case fatality. These calls were a great help to me and to us.

*   *   *

We were satisfied that if we needed to step things up, we knew what to do. It is worth setting out some of the principles and key understandings that informed and guided us.

An effective pandemic response depends on having an agile, flexible, evidence-based approach that is comprehensive, layered and multidimensional. It must consider population measures that may be required as well as measures to protect people who are vulnerable to its consequences. It is based on WHO principles that were well known to us as public health doctors.

At those early night-time meetings, we discussed our preparedness in terms of our systems for disease surveillance, laboratory testing and contact tracing. We would be dependent on the sharing of early information and international risk assessments to enable us to identify the measures we might need to protect high-risk populations, such as the elderly and those with underlying health conditions. We were very clearly focused on how best to put in place clear, trusted, authoritative communication so that we could provide accurate information about the risks and how to prevent infection, as well as updates on the disease, what we knew and did not know and what measures people could take in their own everyday lives.

International advice from WHO and ECDC was also key to our understanding of necessary infection prevention and control measures for preventing the spread of the disease. These measures included, in time, measures we advised on in relation to hand hygiene, wearing masks, social distancing, and isolation and quarantine measures.

Protecting the public from public health threats also requires effective health services for people who may need medical care, isolation and admission. This in turn depends on maintaining the health and wellbeing of the health workforce who will be needed in the provision of health services to the wider public.

Underpinning all of this – and I had a keen sense of the importance of this from my swine flu experience – was our dependence for the effectiveness of our pandemic response on national solidarity, which in turn would require clear leadership and good collaboration and co-ordination among our public health team, the HSE and health service providers, government and its agencies, civil society and other stakeholders.

We had a pre-existing national pandemic influenza plan, which was being updated in the light of the experience of swine flu, but it was taking time and had not been completed. That turned out to be somewhat fortuitous, in my opinion. Covid showed that some countries with advanced and detailed pandemic plans which were based on influenza as the most likely pandemic virus had to 'unlearn' these details and pivot quickly to respond to the realities of Covid-19, which presented very different challenges from influenza.

One of my learnings from all these experiences is the importance of preparedness plans being based on good principles rather than being overburdened by spurious detail which could inhibit rapid adjustment based on the specifics of a given incident.

I also knew we needed to carefully document everything we were doing, with clear agendas and clear minutes of every meeting. When this Covid emergency ended, there would be a need for good documentation to support the learning of lessons. And publishing those records as comprehensively as possible would be key to developing and maintaining public trust.

There was by now an evolving understanding of the transmission potential of this new virus. At the beginning, there was a very strong sense that it was a predominantly lower respiratory tract virus, which might mean it is slightly harder to transmit but people may develop more serious illness as a consequence of it. But this was changing, and we needed to flow with that, leaving room for uncertainties, while at the same time giving as much certainty as we could.

* * *

On 23 January 2020, my sister Breda turned 50 and planned a big party for family and her friends. Clodagh and Ronan and their 12 cousins on the Holohan side of the family always love the get-togethers in Breda's house. I drove down to Limerick for the party with Clodagh, just the two of us. Emer wasn't well enough to come and Ronan had something else on. We went down on a Saturday afternoon and back up on a Sunday, with Clodagh driving – her first time driving a long motorway journey. I sat in the passenger seat, making calls.

There was growing concern by then. A strong sense that this virus was on the move, and we needed to get to a new phase of our preparations. As we drove back on Sunday, I made the decision that it was time to hold the first NPHET meeting.

The design intention of a NPHET is to facilitate public health major emergency planning and response. It brings the key people from organisations who have the relevant authority into one room to have one conversation, as opposed to bilateral conversations, which would be far less efficient.

There had been a NPHET convened on swine flu, and another on an antibiotic resistant organism ('superbug') called carbapenem-resistant enterobacteriaceae (CRE), declared as an emergency in 2017. The CRE NPHET was a tight group of relevant officials and experts in applicable fields.

And then Covid came along. The first Covid NPHET meeting was called for 27 January. At the outset, we met twice a week, sometimes more frequently. Some of the meetings needed to be scheduled at short notice in order to respond to new developments that arose internationally. All members understood the need to prioritise this work at these early stages and were very understanding of the need for short-notice meetings at inconvenient times.

Chairing the NPHET was a major undertaking. There was the singular responsibility for the outcome, to achieve consensus and ensure that was recorded in clear advice to the minister at each point, in a letter to which I could put my name. But there was also the process – how each meeting was managed and how it felt. From the end of March 2020, which was quite early on, all meetings were conducted on Zoom. That brings its own challenges. Building rapport, developing an *esprit de corps*, and being able to 'read the room' are all much more difficult on Zoom. It doesn't lend itself to the open debate that happens in a real room. You have to take points one by one. And when you need to create consensus, it is much slower.

With the number of members we had, in excess of 30, and the detail of the data we had to examine, meetings could be very long. It was a physical challenge as much as anything.

Sitting alone in my office with the door closed for hours at a time and having to be tuned in to what was being said. One thing I found difficult was that the 'chat' function would sometimes be used to make points in parallel and it could at times be difficult to follow that as well as the meeting itself. I asked for people to keep substantive points for the meeting rather than putting them into the chat, and that helped. But I was conscious that we had not agreed a good enough 'rule' around chat at the outset. And I didn't want to change the ground rules midstream.

I had a really strong secretariat team to manage the process of the NPHET. The task of preparing accurate minutes, and ensuring a detailed letter was ready for the minister as quickly as possible after the meeting ended, did not happen by accident. The team would always have a set of agreed actions to show on the screen at the end of each meeting – so everyone would leave the meeting clear on what we had agreed and what would be contained in the letter to the minister.

By late January, we needed to be proactive and open in our communication. We were prepared, and now we needed the public to be informed and prepared. I was confident that Ireland was in a position to hit the ground running. Bad news would come our way for sure in the weeks ahead, and I knew that bad news is best from someone you know and trust. We had to get public trust on our side.

Again using the experience I had gained during the dioxin and swine flu events, I was very focused on the communication message that we needed to convey to the public. After every meeting, I made sure we spent time discussing and planning our bottom line so we could be clear about what message we were intending to get across.

Having the public buy into what we were saying and getting them to trust us wasn't just PR. It was a deliberate instrument of our strategy. Given that this was a new virus, in a population with no immunity, no drugs and no vaccine, the only thing that we had to protect the health and lives of the population was the willingness of the public. We had to engage their hearts and minds in the importance of the task of protecting each other.

Therefore the intention was to focus on the steps people could take to identify their own risks of picking up the infection, the early signs of infection and the signs and symptoms of more serious disease. This would allow people to take measures to protect themselves, and prevent them transmitting it to other people.

We knew even in these early days that fairly extreme measures were being taken in certain countries. There were reports of people being barricaded into their homes and apartment blocks, and of technology being used to monitor people. We couldn't take control measures like these, and obviously I would not have wanted to. But that meant we would have to rely on the public to accept the advice we were giving them of their own volition. They had to want to follow the advice based on their understanding of and trust in what we were telling them in relation to the harm this disease could cause. Trust was the tool we had, and we had to treat it with respect and consideration, because if we didn't have that, we had nothing.

Trust also depended on where the information was coming from. It couldn't be seen to be a political message, because that could create distrust among some sections of the population. It was very important to emphasise that ours was not a political message. As CMO, I therefore led a daily factual press briefing, without involvement from politicians, which would be easily understood and trustworthy so that the general public could take actions that were important in protecting their health.

* * *

Around 30 January, the WHO made a formal declaration that Covid was a public health emergency of international concern (PHEIC). I appeared on *Morning Ireland* the next morning to explain what this meant. At this stage, isolated cases were beginning to appear here and there around Europe, the majority of which had a direct travel link to China or Southeast Asia.

The pattern we expected to experience initially was first a small number of imported cases with direct exposure to China or other regions with higher numbers, followed by more cases and clusters of infection with direct links to other confirmed cases, and ultimately followed by cases and clusters in which no link to either travel or contact with other cases could be identified. What couldn't be known is whether and how quickly we would move through that precise pattern.

Our aim was to maximise the likelihood of picking up a case as soon as it arose, putting in place effective measures to stop that case infecting other people, tracking the contacts of that case and limiting their possibility of becoming cases and transmitting the disease further. The approach at that point was one of so-called containment.

It may be useful to briefly outline what containment and mitigation mean in the context of an unfolding epidemic or pandemic. They are two important strategies in pandemic management and they are aimed at slowing down the spread of a contagious disease and reducing its impact on society. Their effectiveness depends on a variety of factors, including the nature of the disease, the availability of resources, and the level of co-operation from the general public. Containment involves measures aimed at preventing the disease from spreading beyond its initial source. This strategy is most effective during the early stages of an outbreak when the number of cases is relatively low. Containment measures include contact tracing, isolation of infected individuals, travel restrictions, and quarantine measures for those who have been in close contact with infected individuals. This is the approach we followed in the early weeks of the pandemic.

At our press briefing on 11 February 2020, prior to any cases occurring in Ireland, I said the following, which reflected the approach of containment and what we were asking of the public during that 'watchful waiting' phase:

> We remain prepared for a confirmed case of Covid-19 (Coronavirus). The Irish health system is currently operating a containment strategy in line with global practice, and all our efforts are focused on identifying suspected cases as they arise and initiating measures to prevent onward transmission of the virus. The National Public Health Emergency Team continues to co-ordinate response efforts between the Health Service and other government departments and agencies, to ensure a comprehensive response in the event of a confirmed case.
>
> Anyone returning from China in the last fourteen days, and experiencing symptoms associated with Covid-19 (Coronavirus), is instructed to self-isolate and contact the health service via phone or email.

It was important to pursue containment for as long as feasible even though we knew, given the virus's high reproduction number and the increasing number of cases now appearing in other countries, especially in Europe, that at some point we would exceed capacity to fully contain each and every case.

Mitigation, on the other hand, focuses on reducing the impact of a disease once it has already spread widely within a community or population. This strategy is typically used when containment measures are no longer effective due to the high number of cases. At that stage, it makes much more public health sense to concentrate resources not on finding every case, but on slowing transmission as much as possible, protecting people who are most vulnerable and providing services to those who have already picked up the infection.

Mitigation measures may include social distancing, wearing masks, limiting large gatherings and promoting good hygiene practices. Mitigation measures can help to slow down the spread ('flatten the curve') of the disease and reduce the burden on healthcare systems, so that they can better respond to the needs of patients with the infection or who otherwise require healthcare.

In our containment period, we wanted to make sure that people were familiar with the common symptoms of Covid and to encourage those who displayed any such symptoms to come forward as early as possible for a Covid test. We were giving GPs and hospitals all the information we could to generate a good understanding of the early and often subtle symptoms and signs, all designed to maximise the likelihood of picking up a case as early as possible, to limit the extent to which it would spread to others. Our message was 'please do the responsible thing and come forward to be tested and we will ensure your confidentiality.'

For me, this promise of confidentiality and avoiding stigma was an important part of the requests we were making of the public. We were asking people to be highly responsible, to look after themselves and to come forward if they had symptoms. This increased our chances of picking up cases around which we could then isolate in order to limit the spread of the disease to others.

People might be reluctant to come if, for example, they were afraid of being identified and perhaps having their name appearing in the media. And it was a legitimate fear. We had seen at the early stages of SARS and swine flu how keen the media were to identify specific cases. We were reinforcing this message of confidentiality, and at the same time building capacity within the system to test for Covid.

By the end of February about 750 tests had been carried out. All were negative. But even the fact that we were testing people appeared to add to fears about Covid among some people.

* * *

Throughout the weeks from late January to the end of February we were in very close contact with international organisations and other countries. The WHO was a source of regular guidance and advice which we listened to very closely. It had a direct understanding in the early days from its knowledge of the affected areas. The ECDC, based in Stockholm, is the EU expert body in infectious disease control. It carried out risk assessments and provided early learning and advice which was invaluable to us. Ireland has a seat on both the governing body and the scientific advisory committee, which enabled us to have a close dialogue with the ECDC in those early days when information was evolving rapidly.

In spite of the good work that the ECDC and WHO did, I could see the impact of Brexit in European preparedness and response. The UK had and still has very substantial expertise and capacity in public health and infectious disease epidemiology. It had always made a major contribution to the European response and the intelligence capacity of the ECDC. I witnessed closely how it had done so during swine flu. Now the UK was moving in a different direction.

There is no question in my mind that Brexit and the position of the UK throughout much of the pandemic contributed to more fragmentation of the European response than would have been the case if there had been no Brexit. Ireland felt this more than most EU countries due, for example, to the common travel area and our extensive consumption of UK media.

That being said, we had a close and very good relationship with Dr Michael McBride, CMO in Northern Ireland, and his team. Throughout the pandemic we held a regular weekly online meeting with them. When the circumstances demanded, we could meet either more or less frequently. Michael was always willing to share the perspectives from the discussion among the UK CMOs that took place each week. Even if the policy decisions being taken were different from those in Ireland, it was always valuable to share intelligence and perspectives.

Michael and I tried our best over the course of the pandemic to ensure that there was consistency in the approaches being taken across the island of Ireland. For reasons beyond our control, that consistency was not always possible, but I am certain that the very good working relationships between us enabled much more synergy and consistency than we would otherwise have seen.

As we prepared for the certainty of the arrival of cases and waves of infection, we could see that the virus was far too contagious for containment to work for very long. We knew that once we began to see significant community transmission, we would have to focus on measures to slow the progression of the disease. The phrase 'let it rip' was being heard in the media in those February days. It was being advocated by some people, especially in the UK, but it was at variance with public health experience and expertise.

The first line of our defence against a wave of infection was public support for population measures designed to prevent infection and slow the spread of infection. The next line of defence was our system of infectious disease surveillance (i.e. monitoring infection levels), early detection, and containment of cases and close contacts of a confirmed case to limit the risk of further cases in individuals and households. The third line of defence was hospital and ICU services for those who were infected and developed severe infection. The more effective the first and second lines of defence, the better protected people would be from the infection and the better our health service would be protected and available for those who did need it.

We had to ensure as much as we could that we spread the wave of infection out over a period of time. That was the intention behind the 'flatten the curve' message. The number of cases per day and per week had to be minimised. But the main purpose was to protect people from getting severely ill in the first place. Protecting ICU capacity so that our services would not be overwhelmed was the secondary purpose. That would also indirectly protect people in that it would mean ICU capacity would be available for those who did need it.

Many commentators and much of the media completely missed that point. We had a lot of very vocal advocacy from within the health service for ICU and hospital developments, which led to much comment in the media in the early days about numbers of ICU beds. The media focus on 'Why isn't the minister funding more beds?' risked diverting everyone from vital public health services which were significantly underdeveloped relative to what we would need. We had to ensure that the focus on ICU capacity would not be at the expense of improving basic public health measures that could prevent people requiring ICU or hospital services. Of course, both are needed, but the balance needs to be right. If we could stop people getting sick or needing ICU in the first place, that had to be our first priority.

I worried at the time about the risk of the national eye being on the wrong ball. Of course, if we had many more ICU staffed beds, we would have had less pressure on those services and more capacity to cope with severely ill cases. But more beds with more severe cases meant a greater impact on public health. Admitting people to ICU beds because of a respiratory viral infection that could be prevented was absolutely not the right objective. We needed to protect as many people as we could from getting the infection. We could avoid them needing ICU by keeping them infection-free. That was our primary obligation. That was my focus throughout the Covid pandemic.

Some people would later argue that Ireland ended up taking population measures for longer than we might have because we didn't have enough ICU capacity in place, and they would offer that as evidence that we were not properly prepared when the pandemic began. It is true that Ireland had one of the lowest numbers of beds per capita in Europe, but even if we could have doubled the ICU capacity of the country and had had enough ICU beds to manage five hundred people at one time, it would not have materially changed our approach. We would still have done everything we could to prevent people ending up in ICU in the first place.

ICU capacity is in public discourse often measured by numbers of beds, but ultimately the key determinant of ICU capacity is the availability of highly trained and skilled nurses and doctors. That is not something that you can dial up very easily if you don't have enough of those people in the system. And we didn't. That too needed to be addressed, but not at the expense of public health capacity developments. Tracey Conroy and her team in the Department of Health worked closely with HSE colleagues to produce a credible plan, which government approved in 2020, for expansion of ICU capacity that would add more beds to the system over the years of the pandemic and leave our ICU departments in a much better state at the end of the pandemic than at the beginning.

* * *

We had no reason to believe that Ireland and the continent of Europe was going to find ourselves so sharply an epicentre of this disease in the way that later happened. Over the course of February, there were sporadic cases in many countries. We were fully expecting that to happen here and we were prepared.

At the same time, the level of fear was intensifying. We have been criticised by some for using fear or perhaps even inciting it as a tool to maintain compliance with measures that we were recommending at the time and since. It is a criticism I totally reject. We had population survey information continuously available to us that showed the levels of public concern and that people watched our press briefings as a means of addressing their fears.

The reality of that time was that, given the accounts coming from China and, later, northern Italy and elsewhere of severe respiratory illnesses and deaths, there was plenty of reason for people to be concerned. The media were reporting severe infections in otherwise healthy people. Social media as well as some less responsible mainstream media conveyed information in colourful ways that didn't help the levels of fear. We were trying to maintain a sense of calm by providing information that people could understand and trust. And by and large, we were managing to do so successfully.

There still wasn't a great deal of concern politically. The first briefing for newly elected Oireachtas members was given by Dr Ronan Glynn in Buswells Hotel on 20 February 2020, the day the new Dáil first came together. Parliamentary staff of two new members showed up. There were no elected representatives in attendance. That changed quickly. Two weeks later a similar meeting took place in the LH 2000 briefing room in Leinster House. It was well attended, mostly by aides. But Micheál Martin was there and asked detailed questions of the team. I talked very frequently to the top officials in the

Taoiseach's department to keep them in the loop. We still didn't have a case, but it was only a matter of time.

One Saturday evening during this period (I recall there was a national league match that I was watching that I had to abandon) a report came through to me that a plane had landed at Dublin Airport on which there was a passenger with a temperature. The early information was that they had originally come from Wuhan. Somehow that information leaked immediately into the political world, and from there to the media.

The HSE, to its credit, already had a public health team on the ground at Dublin Airport. This is where our forward planning swung into action. This team of public health doctors from the HSE were working hard on a Saturday night to do exactly what our plans provided for. They were systematically going through the list of passengers, with a questionnaire for all of them to fill out. It was clear that at least some people would have to be quarantined, in accordance with the protocol of the time, which is very distressing. But all this meant was that the system was working. An elaborate response was kicking into place. I can't recall how many calls I got that evening over something that to me was evidence of good plans being effectively implemented. Suffice to say the match was well over when the phone stopped ringing, and it was only much later that I found out the result!

The media was all over this. Immediately images appeared online of ambulance service staff in hazmat suits at Dublin Airport, ambulances leaving and going to the Mater Hospital. The Mater was the National Isolation Centre, the most expert centre to which the most serious and unusual infections would be admitted. The initial plan was that presumed and confirmed cases would be admitted there, to limit risk of transmission to others.

There were high levels of concern, even though this was exactly how things were supposed to work. That Saturday evening suspected case at Dublin Airport turned out to be negative. And then, on 29 February, we did get our very first case.

It was, again, a Saturday. Things were getting busier on the work front. We were manning the pumps seven days a week. I hadn't had a day off in weeks. I had received a Christmas present of a voucher for a one-day fish cookery course in Howth Castle Cookery School. I knew I might not get the chance to do the course unless I took it then, so, on 29 February, that's what I did to have a break from the pressure.

The course finished at about four o'clock that Saturday and I went back into the Department to see how things were going. I was going up in the lift to my office when my phone rang. It was Ronan Glynn. 'We have our first case.'

CHAPTER SEVENTEEN
Covid: Our First Case

THE FIRST NPHET PRESS conference took place on Saturday 29 February 2020. It confirmed the first Covid case in this country. We held the press conference in the Department of Health briefing room, rather than Government Buildings.

At that stage, the level of awareness among the public was limited. Up to the point of the first case, our public health messages were focused on recognising symptoms, the need to come forward for testing and the importance of self-isolation. We didn't want to ask the public to adopt measures any sooner than they were needed or have them in place for any longer than they were required.

Deirdre Watters was the head of communications at the Department of Health. She and I came to work very closely in the course of the pandemic. I trusted her advice and that of her team. She was very strongly of the view that maintaining a separate 'identity' for press briefings at the Department of Health would be very important.

I agreed with Deirdre's advice. How right she was. We were both clear that this was about maintaining the public's trust in what we would need to tell them. We knew that might erode over time, and we had to guard it as much as we could.

Covid was new, and so we genuinely had limited insight into what might happen in the months and years ahead. We needed to keep hold of every advantage we had, and public trust was a significant one.

I telephoned the minister to tell him about the case and he decided to come to the Department. I felt very strongly that we needed to ensure that the public health messaging – the advice we would need to give to the public and which we needed them to follow – should come not from the minister but from me as CMO. I believed that we would get much better buy-in as a result. I also knew that the minister needed to clearly communicate his efforts to mobilise resources from government and initiate wider political and multisectoral support. The public health and health service response depended on that wider support and Minister Harris was very successful in that regard.

I anticipated a difficult conversation insofar as I thought the minister might want to have a press response in which we both participated, rather than maintaining separate communications. That evening before the press conference, Minister Harris and I considered the various options and had a very constructive conversation which set an important precedent in keeping the public health and ministerial messages separate for the whole of the course of the pandemic.

There was, as a result, very good alignment between Minister Harris and me throughout his time as minister on this issue. He was very supportive of the public health advice both in public and behind the scenes. I think as a result his standing with the public was strengthened for his remaining months in office as Minister for Health.

Circumstances made it easier for me to have a conversation along these lines with a minister. My length of experience and the range of issues I had dealt with meant I had confidence in myself. I was able to call it as I saw it and was ready to accept that if the minister didn't approve of what I was doing or saying, to the extent that he wanted me to stop or to leave, he just had to tell me or ask me. I wasn't afraid of that.

* * *

Covid was probably a once-in-a-lifetime event. It was obvious from early on that we might need to advise on the introduction of unprecedented population measures that would be very difficult and challenging.

We listened carefully to early advice from the WHO and from the ECDC. We also maintained a close watch on what other countries were doing. At times we were all looking back as far as the Spanish flu in 1918 for an understanding of the measures that might become necessary. Throughout late January and February we worked on updating our preparedness, including consideration of what the specifics would be. During that time, Europe was mostly reporting isolated or small numbers of linked cases.

One early test of the impact of the challenges of this came in late February with the question of a Six Nations rugby match against Italy due to take place in Dublin. The NPHET was of the view that the match should not proceed and advised accordingly. The IRFU (Irish Rugby Football Union) asked for meetings with the government. While they had a very legitimate and reasonable request to discuss the matter, I think the initial tone of response – for us to almost explain ourselves and our data to the IRFU – was unfortunate. Thankfully, the minister and I had a constructive meeting with them and the match did not proceed.

In early March, there was a sudden surge in presentations of severe respiratory infection to hospitals in the north of Italy. The early information about SARS CoV-2, the virus that causes

Covid-19, had showed it had this potential. It was clear that there was widespread community transmission right across the region that had not been fully recognised until it led to a wave of deaths and severely ill people requiring hospitalisation.

I recall the impact of that very clearly. The world took note. Italy's experience was a clear illustration of just how quickly the infection can impact public health, stretch the capacity of a modern healthcare system to breaking point, and lead to many preventable deaths. It was terrifying for the communities who had to live through it, and for those who watched it unfold. This was the first place in Europe to experience such an overwhelming surge in cases, severe illness and deaths. TV screens were showing images of people queuing to be assessed in hospital and having oxygen administered while waiting in the queue. Nothing like this had been seen in living memory in this part of the world.

Italy announced an immediate lockdown of a number of its northern cities in response. The army was on the streets. But it wasn't enough. Because of the lead time between cases in the community and presentations of severe infection to hospital, it would continue to get worse for some time before there was any likelihood of improvement. I knew that if they had such widespread community transmission in Italy, it had the potential to happen anywhere. And sure enough in the coming weeks we saw and heard of how overwhelmed the hospital and ICU system became in London, Madrid, Paris, Brussels and many other western European cities.

It was clear this infection would come to Ireland in significant volumes. We had extensive exposure to community transmission in Italy, through people taking skiing holidays in that part of Europe. We could not aspire to completely prevent it. Through our membership of the EU, we are increasingly legally, culturally, economically and socially integrated with Europe. For many other reasons the same applies to the UK, with which we share a common travel area. There was a lot of talk and some high-level advocacy about 'zero Covid' in those times and the weeks that followed. It was a good example of a phrase that was new to me at the time: magical thinking.

I was very clear in my own mind at this point: The only means of preventing catastrophic impact on mortality, severe illness and enormous pressure on hospital-based services in Ireland was to 'flatten the curve' by maintaining control of community transmission. This meant we had to pick cases up as early as possible, we had to intervene as quickly as possible with control measures, we had to act decisively and we had to keep people with us.

A breakdown in solidarity would have had significant consequences. We needed to maintain trust in our advice. We were trying to refocus the public away from alternative sources of advice on social media and elsewhere. However, by the second week of March, within two weeks of our first case, there were worrying signs of fragmentation in public solidarity. Unilateral decisions and actions were being announced or called for which were not based on public health expertise.

Prominent examples, which were amplified in the media, included calls for individual schools to be closed, and GAA clubs that had begun banning matches. The Nursing Homes Association was calling for visits to nursing homes to be cancelled. We had had no nursing home outbreaks reported at that point and the role of asymptomatic transmission – people without symptoms passing on the virus – was not known. That was soon to change, but at that precise point there had been no such reports.

*   *   *

After that first NPHET press conference on 29 February 2020, we held a daily NPHET press conference to keep the public informed. This enabled us to provide reassurance for the public, who were understandably fearful, given what was being seen in other countries and how it was being characterised in print and broadcast media. We believed our approach would give Ireland a good chance of avoiding the worst impacts of Covid. We wanted the public to hear that message. We therefore focused on the basic and most important measures they could take, such as how to recognise infection, what to do with symptoms, the importance of coming forward for testing, and measures people could take to limit its spread.

Case numbers increased through early March. We announced a new number each day; the total in the 24 hours up to lunchtime on the day of the briefing. This number was therefore made up of all the previous day's positives from lunchtime onwards, added to the morning ones from the day of the press briefing.

I recall a key moment that followed the regular NPHET press conference on 11 March, at which we reported nine new cases, bringing the total to date to 43. We gathered for a short debrief. That was standard practice. Cillian de Gascun was looking at his phone. I heard an expletive. I asked what was up and he told me that the lab had been on to him. There were another 27 positives for that afternoon's testing alone. I can remember the shiver down my spine.

I called a NPHET meeting for later that evening. I didn't need to wait for any more information to tell me that this was the moment we had to act.

* * *

The NPHET meeting began sometime after 9pm that evening. It took place at the Department of Health in the top-floor conference room. While we didn't talk about it in these terms at the time, the NPHET never again met face to face. In fact,

I never physically met a number of the members in the entire course of the NPHET.

We ordered in some food; it would be a long night ahead. A consensus could be the only reasonable outcome if we believed in the importance of trust and solidarity. But that was difficult. It took time. Sometimes a lot of time. But I was very clear that it was important that we reach consensus and record the fact that we did reach it. If we expected the country to unite behind the advice we were providing, surely that placed an obligation on us to unite behind those recommendations. Of course, we needed to debate them. We needed to come to a clear judgement to which we would all be loyal, having had the debate informed by all the perspectives and expertise on the NPHET.

We considered all the emerging data. We considered the steps we should take in light of the ECDC-recommended categories of measures and restrictions as set out in its Guidelines for Non-Pharmaceutical Measures to Delay and Mitigate the 2019-NCOV Impact. We agreed in that meeting on 11 March to recommend a national cessation of visits to healthcare settings, limits on mass gatherings, and also the closure of schools, universities and childcare facilities.

It was well after midnight, the early hours of 12 March, by the time the meeting concluded. Now I needed to brief the minister. With him was Tánaiste Simon Coveney, acting for Leo Varadkar, who was in Washington for the annual St Patrick's Day visit. This was a difficult message for me to have to convey. It was late at night and I was exhausted – we all were. I could never have envisaged being in such completely uncharted territory as CMO. I felt the weight of responsibility in that moment.

I was joined by two colleagues, who were also members of the NPHET, at that meeting, for support and solidarity: Tracey

Conroy and Fergal Goodman, who were friends as well as colleagues. They had policy responsibility for acute hospitals, and primary and community care, respectively; very relevant to the potential impacts of Covid and the nature of preparedness that was in place.

We explained to Minister Harris, Tánaiste Coveney and other colleagues our analysis and the measures we were recommending. That went on until about 2.30am. Minister Harris was keen to ensure we knew that the NPHET had his full support in this challenging situation. The minister and the Tánaiste would have to be part of an unprecedented government decision that much of the country was to shut down its activities. They would be expected to explain it to their cabinet colleagues. They left the meeting to call the Taoiseach in Washington and we waited for their return.

As we concluded, Simon Coveney asked if we had eaten, how much sleep we would get and overall how we were feeling. The intensity of our work over the weeks had been significant, and it had been a long night.

The following morning, 12 March, Leo Varadkar came down the steps of the Irish Embassy in Washington to speak to the nation, 'about Coronavirus and Covid-19'. He announced the measures we had recommended, and the reasons for them; 'We're doing it for each other. Together, we can slow the virus in its tracks and push it back. Acting together, as one nation, we can save many lives.'

CHAPTER EIGHTEEN

Covid: 'The Hammer and the Dance'

THAT FIRST STAGE OF restrictions announced by the Taoiseach on 12 March 2020 was a long way from the full set of measures that were recommended by the NPHET over the following two weeks. We knew we were seeing a fire catch, and that we needed to step on it quickly and decisively.

The recommendations we put forward largely required voluntary compliance. There was no additional legislation in place at that time to enforce them. But there was no sense that we needed that. After that early-hours meeting with Minister Harris and Tánaiste Coveney, my belief was that everyone knew how serious the situation was, and so the public, the political system and the media were primed to expect some significant measures.

I felt that there was confidence in us and what we were doing, both among the public and within the political system. I was grateful for that confidence, and very conscious of the heavy responsibility that had come my way.

Until then, the role of CMO would have been familiar to people in the health system but not among the wider public. Yes, I had been in the media at times, when that was necessary, but now all of a sudden I was in front of the entire country, every evening. Telling people things they would rather not hear. All the while being very aware of the impact this was going to have on lives and communities.

As the weeks progressed, the NPHET started to become a large machine with many subgroups and advisory processes feeding into it. There was a very large number of people involved and many more supporting it all in process terms, ensuring that everything flowed smoothly, clearly and in accordance with the priorities and the evolving understanding of the disease.

The complexity and scale of the NPHET was captured in a diagram in the National Plan published by the government on 16 March 2020. That plan was the product of a very significant programme of work which was mostly carried out by my colleagues in the Department of Health. It was a whole-of-government plan, but in fairness to all my colleagues in the Department, there was no significant mobilising of forces from elsewhere to come and assist the Department throughout the course of the pandemic to implement it. We had to find from within through re-prioritising work. That meant stopping other essential programmes of work in the Department of Health. I think any future system of emergency response must find a means of redirecting government resources quickly and easily to the lead department to support the response.

One of the most important developments to boost our response capacity was in relation to the modelling of disease patterns. I was taking my daily early morning walk in Bushy Park one Sunday in late February or early March, and wondering whether we had enough capacity to model the disease patterns as we might have to. In part I was concerned that we were somewhat reliant and perhaps influenced by UK modelling capacity, which had in the past come in for criticism. I thought we would need something much bigger than the capacity we had in place in the health system. I had an idea. I rang Ronan Glynn from my walk to kick it around. He was used to these early morning calls by now! I wondered whether we could appeal to the best analytical brains in Ireland and have them pull on the green jersey to pool their efforts to help us. Now the idea was a plan.

I rang some key people to see where I might find the best modelling brains in Ireland. First was my sister-in-law Orla Feely, now president of UCD, who was then Vice President for Research and Innovation. She advised me to talk to Brendan Murphy, head of the Mathematics Department in UCD. I called him and he was immediately on board. I then called Philip Nolan. Philip was a classmate from medical school and he and I interned together in St Vincent's. He had been president of Maynooth University for almost 10 years at that time. He was on board too and knew of others who would be certain to help. I could feel momentum building.

I called Liz Canavan, assistant secretary in the Department of An Taoiseach. She was a very long-standing colleague of mine. I knew that an ask from her as a top official in the Taoiseach's Department would be responded to. She therefore reached out to the Economic and Social Research Institute (ESRI) and the Central Statistics Office (CSO). They were on board. Within a few days, we convened a meeting in the Department of An Taoiseach with all of these willing and highly expert volunteers. The task was to build a new pioneering national modelling capacity and process for the purpose of Covid. It needed terms of reference, members to join, a process to operate, and a chair.

Philip Nolan agreed to chair it. Philip made himself available in a fully committed way over the course of the pandemic to build a team of the best analytical brains in Ireland to model the disease and its patterns to inform all the advice and decisions that would be made over the coming years. The members of that team gave of their time selflessly and in a spirit of true public service. They were unfairly criticised for 'getting it wrong', including by many who would and should have known better, but it did not deflect them from their work. They published their minutes in full and made their models available for public scrutiny.

As head of the modelling team, Philip worked very closely with me and my core team. He was part of every NPHET, frequent internal meetings and the daily press briefings. He, along with Ronan Glynn and me, attended Covid oversight meetings chaired by the Secretary General of the Department of An Taoiseach Martin Fraser, the cabinet committee meetings, and many other meetings along the way. I remember walking down the stairs in the Department of the Taoiseach with Philip as we made our way out after a Friday afternoon meeting with the Taoiseach, Tánaiste, and ministers and secretaries general. We recalled walking along corridors together as interns in St Vincent's and wondered if we could in our wildest imagination have ever seen where we would end up together.

*   *   *

At times, some commentators implied that those of us on the NPHET who carried these responsibilities and who were advising on these decisions were people who didn't live in the real world. It was as though, for some, we existed in a bubble that kept us separate from reality.

That was far from the truth. My family was impacted just as everyone was. Emer, already isolated because of her illness, was going to be even more so. She wouldn't be able to see her parents, siblings or friends. Her world was shrinking even further. The measures that would keep her safe from the disease that would shorten her life would cut her off from direct physical companionship at a time when she needed it more than ever.

Ronan was in fifth year and Clodagh was in her first year at university. They too were going to live the consequences of what we recommended. There were different difficulties for different age groups, but there is no doubt that young people were heavily impacted. Almost everything at that age – school, study, sport, friendships, relationships, travel – is social. And all these pursuits were being restricted and placed out of reach for that generation. At their age, that period represented a large proportion of their lives.

We knew we needed to recommend these very difficult measures, such as restricting social contacts in all sorts of settings, but we didn't have certainty as to how long they would be required. The emphasis of people on the NPHET was on what we needed to do, now, to get back in control of community transmission. We believed this would flatten the curve to levels that our public service and especially the health system could manage and buy as much time as possible in the hope that at some point new vaccines or treatments might come on stream.

There was a phrase used a great deal at the time – 'the hammer and the dance'. This was a metaphor that described different approaches to managing the spread of the virus: strict measures (the hammer) would be implemented, then eased for a time (the dance), then reimplemented and eased as necessary in a continuous cycle. What was unclear was how long each of those phases would or could last. And how long public support would remain.

Some commentators were expounding on these issues with great certainty, something no one could have had. Among them were people who should have known better, given their professional backgrounds. Those of us who held actual responsibility for how we should respond rarely expressed such certainty. We could hope, we could estimate, we could monitor, but there were simply too many variables to be certain about how this would run its course and how long that would take. Complex problems do not have simple solutions.

We were confident that we could get to a point of control if we limited transmission opportunities across the population. But we knew that as soon as we lifted restrictions, the conditions would re-emerge for viral transmission. And yet we also knew that, in the times when we had limited levels of transmission, it wasn't proportional to maintain the very heavy restrictions . . . It was a constant dynamic between these things. Population measures had to be applied no earlier than necessary, and for no longer than necessary.

* * *

After those first measures and restrictions were introduced, Covid cases and their impact continued to increase. There was very definitely an element of trial and error in the early days. We couldn't say for sure that the first set of measures would work in such a way as to obviate the need for further and more aggressive measures. They didn't. Cases continued to rise – to above 1000 – and our ICU numbers increased significantly. So much so that the NPHET issued further recommendations to the government on 24 March aiming to damp down continued transmission.

That second set of measures recommended by the NPHET was approved immediately by the government. These included measures relating to hospitality, leisure activities and mass gatherings. Thankfully, government was on board and supportive of our advice and how it was formulated and presented, and so were the media. My recollection is that there was no significant dissent at this point from what we were recommending.

That was to prove important as very soon after the second set of measures it became clear from our close monitoring that we would need to go further. By 24 March, we had seen in excess of 1800 cases, ICU admissions had roughly doubled to 71 and there had been 19 deaths. We would need every possible measure in place to regain some control of the widespread community transmission. This was driving a rapid increase in our ICU admissions. We had to avoid what had happened in northern Italy, London, Paris, Madrid and elsewhere. We were running out of time.

On Friday 27 March we recommended a third set of measures to be implemented immediately. These included strict stay-at-home measures and limited all but the most essential work and activities. Government agreed to our advice but there wasn't quite the same unquestioning acceptance. There was definitely some querying of why we were back so soon, only three days after the second set of measures was agreed. 'Should we not wait and see if the previous measures are working?' was one question.

I had to answer those questions clearly and comprehensively, by explaining 'this is how the virus has moved, this is what we're seeing, so this is how we're responding.' There were many important things we did not yet know about SARS CoV-2 and Covid – and we were open about that. However, there is real danger in delaying what is necessary because you don't yet know the answer to every single question.

To the question, 'Can we not wait until next week?', my short answer was 'No'. To wait until the following cabinet meeting on the 31 March would have been four more days of transmission, and each day mattered. In simple terms, the combination of high reproduction number (the average number of cases that result from each case) and a short generation time (the average time between each 'generation' of new infections), as with SARS CoV-2, would, without measures to prevent it, lead to exponential growth which could suddenly overwhelm us, as we had seen elsewhere in Europe. We needed every control measure in place and we needed them urgently in order to prevent this.

It can be difficult to understand and predict exponential growth, because we think in a linear fashion. If you asked most people if you started with €1 and doubled what you have every day, how long it would take to reach €1 million, their answer is almost never right. In fact, it takes less than 21 days to get from €1 to €1 million. That is exponential growth and the human mind almost always underestimates it.

I remember participating in the press conference to announce these measures with the Taoiseach and the minister. I recall standing outside Government Buildings beside the beautiful fountain, doing a live interview to explain all of this on the nine o'clock news. That was the point at which we went into 'lockdown', as it became known. It was a cold March evening. Above all, I remember walking back with Deirdre to the Department of Health, past all the lovely pubs, and wishing it was a different time and that we could pop in to warm ourselves with a Friday evening tipple.

* * *

This was a time of unprecedented uncertainty. The global scientific community was still learning. Scientific knowledge was growing and at times changing very rapidly. The first half of 2020 saw over 20,000 research publications related to Covid, almost 10,000 pre-print articles, the initiation of hundreds of new clinical trials and extensive collaboration and data sharing. It is not surprising in this context that on some important questions there was not always a settled body of opinion. That is why it was important to maintain openness and readiness to change advice in response to new evidence and in particular the guidance of expert international bodies such as the WHO and the ECDC.

One strength of Ireland's pandemic response in the face of this surge of new evidence, research and data relating to Covid was the creation of a strong evidence synthesis function to support the work of the NPHET and its expert advisory group. Evidence synthesis is an expertise that combines information from multiple studies investigating the same topic to comprehensively understand their findings. This work was led by Máirín Ryan, deputy CEO of HIQA. Over the course of the pandemic, Máirín and her team produced and published on HIQA's website many detailed pieces of advice, assessments of evidence and of international practice which were of the highest standard and were often cited by ECDC in its own advice and guidance.

Cillian de Gascun was a key member of the team – I trusted and valued his judgement fully. He is a virologist of international standing and was fully plugged into the unfolding international understanding of this new virus. SARS CoV-2 was a brand-new virus that was still adapting to humans as a host, and changing as it did so. We have seen the various mutations that have resulted. We expected these could occur, of course, but we didn't know the timing or form any new variant would take. Through the pandemic, Cillian kept us expertly up to date with new variants and mutations. The world has to keep monitoring to enable these changes to be rapidly detected so that appropriate measures can be implemented.

A critical feature of infection from SARS CoV-2 is that some people are infectious for up to two days before they develop symptoms. Another is that people can be infectious even with mild or no symptoms. Pre-symptomatic and asymptomatic transmission made control of the pandemic more difficult because measures based only on symptomatic individuals were less effective. This was a key consideration in recommending unprecedented social distancing measures to minimise the spread of Covid-19.

A simple rule of thumb with a new virus, which does not always hold true, is that as new strains appear over time, they tend to become more transmissible but less severe. After all, it is not in the evolutionary interest of a new infectious organism to kill its host. In virological terms, the virus develops more effective means of transmitting if it makes people ill but doesn't kill them; that helps it to survive and thrive.

Initially, we did not know precisely how serious an infection this was at the population level, even if it was clear from the early Wuhan experience that some individuals could have severe and fatal outcomes. The more severe cases of a new infection will be the first to come to the attention of health services and be recorded, much more so than very mild versions of the infection. A disease that is new is more easily picked up if it causes people to become seriously ill or to die. Serious illness and deaths quickly come to the attention of hospitals and health authorities. Mild symptoms cause less concern, present less frequently to health services and are therefore not as likely to be recorded. This means that it takes time for relevant studies and observations to pick up the true patterns of mild and more severe infection.

There was also considerable uncertainty about transmission by those who are asymptomatic relative to those who are symptomatic. Asymptomatic transmission of SARS CoV-2 refers to the spread of the virus by individuals who are infected but do not show any symptoms. Symptomatic transmission occurs when individuals with SARS CoV-2 who have symptoms, such as coughing or sneezing, spread the virus to others. In those early days, while there were many claims, hard evidence from well-designed studies was more limited.

There was much passionate debate about the use of masks in the early days. An important means of transmission of Covid is via droplets released while talking, coughing, laughing or sneezing. Masks act as a barrier to these droplets, prevent and contain droplet release and can help to protect the wearer from contracting the virus. Real-world observations of mask use show that countries that mandated and encouraged their use have generally had lower rates of Covid-19 transmission than those that have not.

The importance of different mechanisms of transmission of SARS CoV-2 was also in dispute. Airborne transmission can be an important source of infection in settings such as indoor spaces, places with poor ventilation, and crowded environments. The relative importance of mechanisms of transmission depends on many factors, such as how much virus a person is shedding, the duration and closeness of contact with others, and the effectiveness of preventive measures such as appropriate use of masks, hand hygiene, physical distancing and indoor ventilation.

There was also considerable focus in the early days on the idea that Covid would die down in summer. That was not an unreasonable expectation. Seasonality is a phenomenon that is seen with many respiratory viral infections. However, 2020 was much too early for patterns of seasonality to be known or assumed.

It was through pooling observations and data at a European and international level – work undertaken by international organisations such as the WHO and the ECDC – that we developed our understanding of the virus, its effects and how best to prevent its impact.

The uncertainty did not diminish the need for good-quality advice to be provided to the public which could be understood, effectively implemented and monitored and ultimately relied upon. A key part of our process in this regard was a meeting called the Medical Leaders' Forum, comprising our core team together with around two dozen or so of the top health professionals and leaders from around the country. This met on a Saturday morning for many months during the first wave. All its meetings bar the first were online. That first meeting was held in a socially distanced fashion on St Patrick's Day 2020 in the press conference room of the Department of Health. There was a palpable sense of togetherness in the room, which gave everyone confidence.

The data might have been uncertain and evolving; there may have been debate about the best responses. But the overwhelming sense I had from this group and the wider medical profession at the time was that everyone bought into the national response and the importance of coming together in solidarity. Minister Harris was a regular attendee, which was appreciated by all the members. The Taoiseach also attended on several occasions. That really helped to maintain a strong sense of the support for the medical community from the political system, and vice versa. It really made a constructive contribution to the solidarity of our national response.

Once the final set of measures were implemented in late March 2020, we knew it would take at least a week to see a positive change in the number of cases. Most of the infections that would come to notice in the following week had already been exposed and were going to go on to develop infection, irrespective of new control measures. Similarly, it was going to take a period of time before the rise in new ICU admissions would start to slow and ultimately fall. The next two weeks of ICU admissions would come from those already infected. Finally, the outcome that would take the longest to show a positive impact would be mortality.

ICU numbers continued to climb well into April 2020. The peak number was about 160 people with Covid in ICU. That meant our ICUs were under significant pressure, which had forced the cancellation of major surgical procedures. However, unlike many other European countries and cities, they were not overwhelmed. And that is a tribute to the solidarity shown by Irish people in following public health advice and also to the professionalism and commitment of the staff in the health service and, in this case, particularly in the intensive care units. Committed. Dedicated. Expert. Fearless.

Once we began to see the positive impact of the measures we had recommend on case numbers, admissions and deaths, the question of 'What next?' arose. 'What is the pathway out of this?' I wished that pathway would be easier and more near-term than I feared it would be.

Vaccines were a long way down the road – that was our belief in the first wave. While we knew that intensive research and innovation efforts were under way around the world, in the spring and early summer of 2020 it just wasn't a realistic thing to be talking about. Yes, we would need to be ready to implement mass vaccination programmes when the time came, but in those early days, that seemed like a faraway dream. We kept an eye on what was happening with these developments, of course, and as time went by, more and more concrete reports came our way which gave us reason to hope. But even then, we remained cautious.

We had some very interesting conversations about whether coronavirus vaccines would be technically possible or whether they would be effective. For the time being, I saw that as being an interesting conversation – nothing more. We would have to wait to see what would emerge from the enormous research and development efforts that were under way to develop a vaccine. And by wait, I really mean get on with the measures we did have available to us and make the best use of them.

* * *

Within a very short space of time in March 2020, we had recommended the cessation of everything except essential retail and essential public services such as health services. We had good reason to believe these measures would be effective. But we couldn't be certain how long it might take and how much things would improve. Another factor yet to be understood was how much people would reduce their adherence to public health guidance as the perception of the risks from this virus diminished.

I don't like the word lockdown. At the time, I never used it and I always advised others not to do so. There is no standard definition of what constitutes a lockdown. In some countries, lockdown might mean your door is bolted shut and you are physically prevented from leaving your home. In other countries the army and police were on the streets in a physical show of force which was often heavy-handed. In yet other places, it meant electronic surveillance of a kind that simply would not be possible or desirable in a free and democratic country.

In Ireland, it meant something much more self-imposed. The restrictions were something that the public bought into. They could not have worked without a very high level of solidarity across the whole population, society and the economy.

The Gardaí were largely sensitive in how they carried out their role during Covid. Their approach was less about the physical imposition of rules and much more about supporting and enabling people to maintain our collective response. We had high levels of compliance from well over 90 per cent of the public. If I could put my finger on what made our response in Ireland so much better from a public health point of view than most of our European neighbours, that would be it.

What was required was for most of the people to follow most of the advice most of the time. We weren't expecting perfection. From the outset, there were media stories of breaches – a gathering in a GAA club or a party in the suburbs, for example. But in public health terms, one event in one location wasn't significant. As indicators of public sentiment, it was useful to keep an eye on such happenings – and I'm not condoning these failures of compliance – but from a public health point of view, they weren't alarming when the context was one where the vast majority of people were complying.

For me, there was too much intolerance of these understandable and often isolated examples of non-compliance. Social media was very focused on identifying individuals who broke lockdown and outing them, but I felt that was the wrong approach. This virus was twice as transmissible as influenza. And we don't succeed in preventing transmission of influenza. We don't hold people individually culpable for the spread. We try to encourage them to be responsible, but we accept that we can't all be perfect all the time.

We tried to encourage a sense of solidarity and responsibility. We were concerned about issues which occurred that threatened erosion of solidarity where breaches concerned public figures. That was a very different matter because it really did undermine solidarity and the sense that we were all in it together.

That said, one of the things I was very clear about behind the scenes was the importance of those of us in prominent leadership positions in the NPHET being obsessive about our personal observation of public health guidance. And it paid off. There were no incidents that I know of in which we NPHET members were identified as not following the advice.

Within a couple of weeks of the third and final set of restrictions being implemented in March 2020, we began to see a positive impact on case numbers.

One thing that we tried to focus on at the time was the fear people clearly felt about attending hospital, even in situations where they needed to. We tried to explain that it was safe to go to the emergency department: 'If you've got something that is worrying you, deal with it as you would have previously.' People were very concerned. Understandably.

Many cases of Covid were picked up in hospital environments, notwithstanding very clear and well-worked-out arrangements put in place to limit that. You cannot fully sanitise hospitals. In fact, one of the dangers of hospitals is the infection risk posed by healthcare-associated infections. Sometimes these are transmitted from patients to staff and sometimes vice versa. There are particular risks where healthcare staff are coming in and out of work while living in the community. In that scenario, it is impossible to completely protect the hospital-dwelling population. Similarly with nursing homes. If there is widespread, uncontrolled community transmission, healthcare workers who live in that community inevitably risk bringing that the infection with them. It is simply impossible to prevent infection, especially where asymptomatic transmission plays an important role, from entering institutions when there is widespread and uncontrolled transmission taking place in the wider community.

As of 27 March, we had measures in place that we believed would lead to control of community transmission. It was appropriate then to give full attention to the question of additional measures focused on vulnerable populations living in institutions.

At the NPHET meeting on 31 March, we recommended a number of significant actions designed to protect residents in long-term residential settings, including nursing homes. These were contained in a detailed paper entitled 'Enhanced Public Health Measures for Covid-19 Disease Management – Long-term Residential Care (LTRC)'. The minister also established an independent panel, chaired by Professor Cecily Kelleher of UCD, to recommend further measures aimed at protecting vulnerable people in these settings.

We were concerned about risks that made protection more difficult than might have been anticipated. For example, there appeared to be a high degree of mobility among agency-employed staff who worked across several nursing homes. Many such staff are low-paid workers, many of whom were living in crowded conditions and in some cases sharing with workers from other sectors such as the meat-processing industry.

We had to try to get to grips with these risks, while also being very conscious of not doing or saying anything that would lead to these workers being 'blamed'. The HSE sought to provide living quarters for people who were working in nursing homes as a way to protect them from the conditions of community infection. But that is a far from simple task.

The sad reality is that we did have a significant wave of infection affecting nursing homes, and with quite high mortality rates in some of those settings. The country was gripped by an infection that has a predilection for vulnerability. If we had set about designing a model of care for older people that was focused on placing them at the greatest possible risk of the serious effects of a respiratory virus such as Covid, we couldn't have done a better job than building and operating the nursing home model that we have.

This was something that every other country with similar models of nursing home care also experienced. We are still a relatively young population compared with Italy, for example, where the proportion of the population aged over 65 is double what it is here. This significantly older population is one of the reasons Italy experienced high mortality. Italy has a large nursing home sector, and experienced very high mortality in that sector.

This is something that has to be tackled in the future. The elderly are still among the most vulnerable population to Covid and to respiratory viral infection in general. Their vulnerability to Covid has been significantly reduced by the impact of the vaccinations, but there is only so much the vaccine can do to protect them. As long as this is our model of care, we are open to another serious infection that disproportionately affects elderly people.

* * *

Throughout those initial months, there was a constant need for decisions to be taken, recommendations to be made, evidence to be weighed and considered. And there was no possibility, ever, of taking much time with these. There was no way you could say, 'I'm going to sleep on this', 'I'm going to take 24 hours and consider this.' I had to keep moving, keep making decisions, keep pace with the evolving situation in which new issues arose almost every day.

In some sections of public discourse, we were criticised for making recommendations without care or regard for or even understanding of the impact on mental health. This was never the case. We knew there would be a serious impact. Many people with mental health issues are also vulnerable to Covid because of pre-existing conditions. There was also the added concern that Covid infection threatened continuity of services on which so many people with mental health illness or other vulnerabilities depend. From the outset we were thinking about issues such as the risks around domestic violence. We thought about risks arising from the decision to close schools, knowing that for some children school is respite.

Our primary responsibility from a public health point of view was to ensure that we gave advice and guidance that would protect the public from picking up this infection in the first place. We knew that Covid presented a substantial exist-ential and preventable risk to their health and the health services upon which they depended. We made public health assessments in the knowledge that there might be unintended or undesirable consequences. Every decision you make has consequences. We couldn't become paralysed by indecision. We were trying to make reasoned assessments of the risk and put in place proportional recommendations to address these risks.

I don't think that doing otherwise would have been right or responsible.

CHAPTER NINETEEN
Covid: Day to Day

DURING THE EARLY MONTHS of the pandemic, something divisive entered public discourse that I greatly disliked. It was a 'Who is actually dying and how much do their lives matter?' line of questioning. I remember a similar question during the swine flu pandemic where questions were raised after we reported a death along the lines of: 'Did the person have underlying medical conditions?' And if the answer to that was 'Yes', there was a sense of 'That's okay then.'

I thought that was despicable.

Vulnerable people with 'underlying medical conditions' were part of our community too. That category included Emer. It included my parents and my parents-in-law, and many people's parents and in-laws. Many people living with chronic illness or aged over 80 are hale and hearty and valuable members of society.

The idea that there were some deaths that were 'okay' goes against everything in my training and my beliefs as a public health doctor. We were never going to be able to completely prevent mortality from an infection as severe as Covid. But the idea that those who were genuinely vulnerable to the severe effects of the disease should be treated as though their lives mattered less was ugly.

What was arising was a sense of 'I'm 20; my risk from this is very low, but my life has been taken away from me and my mental health is impacted as a result.' If one looks at it from the point of view of an individual, that case could be made. But the strength of Ireland's pandemic response was based on whole-population solidarity. That means everybody participated in the societal effort to limit transmission, even if the beneficiaries of that were likely to be a defined group – such as the elderly and those with underlying conditions. That is the kind of society we choose to live in.

Each successive wave of infection over the course of the pandemic was characterised by early transmission among young people followed by transmission in older age groups where mortality was much higher. That reflects how society functions. Social contact is greater among the young. It is a simple demographic and epidemiological fact, not a reason to assign blame to young people.

In the main, Ireland had good compliance, even though, understandably, that eroded over time. In the beginning, most people were reasonably content to do as the public health advice recommended. We used a twice-weekly population survey to measure public attitudes, ideas, concerns and expectations. It also asked about compliance with key aspects of our advice. We could see that over time people found the restrictions more and more frustrating. This increasing disquiet also began to emerge in political circles and in the media.

Questions increasingly asked of the minister in the Dáil, or of me and my colleagues in our NPHET press briefings, sometimes felt like an attempt to 'catch us out'. For example, there were questions about apparent inconsistencies in the public health advice. 'Why leave pubs open in hotels, but close them in the community?', 'Why is it okay to have a burger with your pint, but it is not okay to just have a pint?' 'The virus doesn't know I'm having my dinner' was the kind of ostensibly witty challenge we received.

The explanation for these 'inconsistencies' was widely misunderstood. It might appear, for example, that allowing hotel residents to have bar service and restaurant meals was inconsistent with closure of non-hotel pubs and restaurants. But the measure had nothing to do with the risk of drinking in a hotel bar compared to a regular bar. Rather, the rationale was that it would result in far fewer social contacts in which transmission was possible than if every pub and restaurant in the country was open. It was a simple measure to reduce the total volume of social contact at the population level.

The '€9 meal' received particular attention in public commentary. In fact, the NPHET did not come up with this. There was legislation already in place for another purpose that was creatively used to enable a distinction between a pub that also had significant restaurant services, and one that did not. Of course, we knew that some people would order a burger and pay €9 for it, not eat it but spend an evening drinking beer instead. Some observers seemed to enjoy pointing those stories out – 'Man Outwits Public Health Advice by Drinking 10 pints and Not Eating a Burger!'

But the value of the measure was that most people did not do that. The great majority of people listened to our advice and followed the spirit of it. That is why it had a positive public health impact.

* * *

The daily press conferences were a vital part of our strategy of clear communication and messaging. They were also a considerable demand on my time and energy. I had to be switched on, ready and properly prepared. In that environment, in front of television cameras and microphones, you're only ever a step away from something going very wrong. A question that can't be answered, or is answered incorrectly, can lead to all sorts of trouble. I always tried to remember that I was speaking not to the journalists in the room but, through them, to people watching at home, listening in cars or on their evening walk who wanted a clear message they could understand and incorporate into their daily lives.

Each briefing was preceded by the 'EpiCall'. This was a Zoom meeting of about 15 key people from the HPSC, the NVRL and the Department of Health which took place around 4pm, seven days a week. They were great people to work with. These were people I relied on and trusted completely. We got to know each other very well, forging the kind of bonds that I imagine are forged in battle. That helped us all personally at a very intense time in our lives. It certainly helped me.

The EpiCall would examine all available data, modelling projections and the relevant facts of the day. It looked at the issues in the same systematic way over the course of that call every day: What was the international information update on vaccines? What was happening in the country? Any pressure points that were building? What was being said in the medical literature? What was being advised by international bodies? Where were the disease dynamics at? We would always conclude with a discussion about the press matters of the day: What are the key issues? What are our messages?

One of the press team would prepare a statement informed by the EpiCall. I would read it, add to it and approve it before the press conference. The final task was to inform the minister of the new data or facts for the day so that he would hear them before the press briefing. That was the daily routine. I always went into the press briefing feeling prepared.

The NPHET meeting was where our policy advice to government was generated. It took place twice weekly or weekly as the prevailing epidemiological situation demanded. I had confidence in the people involved and the process of the NPHET. It was the subject of much scrutiny and of criticism over the course of the pandemic from its first meeting in late January 2020 to its final meeting on 17 February 2022. That final meeting was the one in which it recommended that it be stood down because it advised that the emergency phase of the pandemic in Ireland had come to an end.

Over the course of the pandemic, the NPHET grew. People were added to provide additional relevant expertise, and a small number were added at the request of the minister in late 2020. The NPHET, including all the groups reporting to it, was a major source of expertise and advice and probably involved in total over two hundred people, all focused on supporting the national response. I was also conscious that many experts were included in the expert advisory group to the NPHET, which was a very important source of advice and analysis of the evidence, and in that way were very much part of the process.

In the earlier stages we had several ad hoc meetings of the NPHET, usually because of a change in disease patterns or significant new information or international advice. Over time, as understanding of the infection increased, meetings took place less frequently.

Both Simon Harris and later Stephen Donnelly, as Ministers for Health, asked to join a NPHET meeting. Each time, I could readily understand their desire to do so. But I was aware, through many experiences with many ministers, that when a minister is in the room, people change what they say. Sometimes they might withhold something more negative or more 'honest' that they wouldn't want a minister to hear; alternatively, they might over-reach in how positively they express something in an effort to impress the minister.

I needed to be in a position where I could trust what I was hearing. And the advice I was giving needed to be independent. In order to trust and stand over the advice that the NPHET was creating and providing to the minister, it was necessary that the minister not be in the room where part of the process that formulated that advice was undertaken.

* * *

In this country the vast majority of the medical community were supportive and all played a significant role in helping our national response. The model of clinical leadership fostered through the HSE clinical programmes really showed its worth during these times. The community of intensive care physicians and their nursing and paramedical colleagues come to mind, as do ambulance staff and staff in nursing homes and similar places. Very often these staff delivered services in spite of their very real fear for their own health and that of their families. I am particularly proud of the response of our GP community and how they rose to the challenge of the pandemic and the vaccination programme. Innovations such as 'GP Buddy' provided valuable real-world data that informed our response at the national level. It was a clear example of leadership and is a credit to the GPs who developed it.

There were some who were advocating 'zero Covid', a policy about which I had serious reservations. Some of its advocates took it upon themselves to write formally to the Minister for Health. I found that particularly undermining. There was also increasing receptiveness in the media to experts who dissented from the mainstream.

CHAPTER TWENTY

Covid: The End in Sight

THE MEASURES IMPLEMENTED IN March had established good population control of the infection in April and May and on into June 2020. There was a plan in place called 'The Roadmap for Reopening Society and Business', drawn up largely by the NPHET and approved by government, which provided a framework for gradually lifting restrictions based on public health considerations and progress in controlling the spread of the virus. It consisted of five stages of escalation and de-escalation in the measures in place to respond to Covid. Each stage reflected factors such as case numbers, hospitalisations and vaccination rate and determined the corresponding restrictions. An updated plan was published in February 2021 called 'Resilience and Recovery: The Path Ahead'.

We began to step down restrictions from 18 May 2020 in line with the roadmap. It provided for minimum three-week intervals between each set of measures. These intervals were to provide sufficient time for changes to take effect, and to gauge whether we were changing too quickly or too slowly.

When we observed that the incidence of the disease continued to drop after the second of these two phases we recommended that the remaining three three-week stages be reorganised into two stages. This was evidence of our commitment to recommend removal of restrictions just as speedily as we recommended their introduction.

At the time, some people were nervous that we were moving too quickly. There was a narrative of 'Oh, that's the government putting pressure on them to open up.' It wasn't. The initiative to speed up the removal of restrictions came from the NPHET. Members of the NPHET didn't enjoy restrictions any more than anybody else in the population. Our lives were curtailed in the same ways as everyone else's, so when the evidence showed that we could remove restrictions, that's what we recommended.

* * *

For those of us who had prominent roles in the NPHET, there was a particular onus on us to follow the guidelines to the letter. We felt the responsibility of that very keenly. As did our families.

Clodagh and Ronan were the most exemplary of observers. Not because of the position I was in, but because they understood Emer's vulnerability. Emer faced some unavoidable exposure. There were many cases in St James's Hospital all through Emer's final year of life. That was a source of major concern and worry for her. However, she had no choice but to attend hospital for treatment at regular intervals. Outside of hospital, she saw no one except me and the children. Given how we lived our lives to protect her as much as possible, St James's Hospital was the place where she was most likely to pick up the infection.

For much of the last year of Emer's life, our children were at home with Emer almost all the time. If not for the pandemic, they would have been out and about, at school, college, playing sport or with friends. And Emer would have wanted it that way. She would never have allowed them to take time away from their lives to be with her. That is just not how she was. She would never have wanted them to stay at home because of her.

The pandemic brought isolation and a reduction in social engagement to everyone. But it allowed Emer and the children an intense period of time together. I was working almost constantly. Clodagh and Ronan really stepped into adult roles, caring for Emer in her everyday life. Clodagh had passed her driving test prior to the pandemic, and was able to bring Emer out for drives. They would sometimes go to McDonald's drive-through, come home and watch *The Great British Bake-Off* together. She looks back on that as one clear 'adult' thing she did to help Emer directly.

Emer never developed Covid. She lived in fear of contracting the virus. And Clodagh and Ronan were almost equally afraid they would pass it to her. So, they remained in close company in their own little bubble. They didn't see their friends. Clodagh had a boyfriend at the time, and she hardly saw him for months. They would talk on the phone, and sometimes he'd come to the gate and she'd talk to him in the garden.

This was absolutely necessary, but also – looking back – it was time together Emer and the children would never have otherwise had during Emer's final year of life.

*   *   *

Coming into that summer of 2020, the case numbers were low (fewer than 10 per day), and Emer was very ill. She had been readmitted to the hospice after a brief hospital admission, and her team were very concerned about her. I realised I was needed at home more than at work. Emer's illness was something that wasn't known about publicly at all before this point.

As it happened, on Stephen Donnelly's first day in office as Minister for Health, I called in to his office, which was practically next door to mine. This was my first face-to-face professional contact with Minister Donnelly in his new role. I told him that I would very shortly have to take a step back for personal reasons. I had known the new Taoiseach, Micheál Martin, since his time as Minister of Health and had a high regard for him, so I also informed him. I had had many conversations with him during the first phase of the pandemic. I knew he understood public health. He had a better grasp of the pandemic than most politicians. I explained my situation to each of them, and how ill Emer was. I didn't know when I would be back. In my mind, I thought Emer was not likely to survive this admission. And so, with the pandemic under very good control, I left. I really didn't know what the future held for my family and me.

On Thursday 2 July 2020, I made the announcement at the daily press conference, and I stepped back immediately. Ronan Glynn took over. Some management board colleagues in the Department of Health took on unrelated parts of my portfolio so that Ronan could focus fully on the pandemic.

Neither Emer nor I was remotely prepared for the scale of response to my announcement. There was prominent coverage in newspapers, on every news bulletin, on Twitter and throughout social media. I was compelled to read them from the perspective of: What would Emer think? What would Clodagh and Ronan think? Those who didn't write about her as though she was already dead wrote as though she had barely any time left. I had to explain to the children that these commentators didn't understand the nature of palliative care and were getting it wrong. Norma O'Leary, her palliative care consultant, was immediately concerned for Emer in the midst of all of that. As was I. And for the children. It was very difficult and unsettling for all of us.

Nothing prepares you for such a situation, living a life that has become highly public, simply because of the job you're doing. Or, in Emer's case, because of who you are married to. The reports and commentary read like obituaries. That had a very negative effect on her emotionally. Emer was not about to give up and submit to her illness.

After the initial media response, there was a second wave – a public response. And that was different. We received an enormous outpouring of letters, cards, emails, texts and social media messages. And the focus of that was people writing *to* Emer, not about her. People expressed admiration and support for her and the way she had lived with her illness and the dignity of how she had responded to it. I particularly recall a lovely letter from a nun in Roscommon who had recently been diagnosed with myeloma. She wrote about how she found hope and inspiration in the knowledge that Emer had lived so long with her illness. Some expressed gratitude for the way Emer had enabled me to do my job, and the role she played in everything that I did.

Emer felt this outpouring as support and warmth. The feeling that people wished her well and hoped for the best for her meant so much to her. It made her feel that there were many people out there who were good and kind and concerned for her.

We never managed to respond to all those letters and messages, but I still hope to do so one day (although lots of people contacted us anonymously). I would like those people who took the time and trouble to be in touch to know how much the kindness of strangers meant to us.

* * *

For the summer of 2020, I focused on Emer and on home. My family needed my full attention during this time. At first it was visits in and out of the hospice, usually twice or three times

206

daily, and maintaining a sense of normality as much as possible with that routine for Clodagh and Ronan, who were by now on summer leave from school and college.

I knew that I couldn't and shouldn't try to do the job from a distance and so I wasn't looking over the shoulders of my colleagues. However, in August and September, it was clear from the rising case numbers that things were heading in the wrong direction. Winter was beginning to loom, when the conditions that facilitate transmission would be more common and when the health system traditionally faced its greatest seasonal challenge. That worried me.

Emer had rallied again, as she did so many times, and was doing much better by late summer. Schools were open and life had returned to some kind of normality for many people. And a big part of 'normal', from Emer's point of view, was me being at work. The doctors were telling her that she had done really well after the most recent hospice admission. She had responded well to radiation for a lesion in her lower back, and to pain relief, and so we talked about how we would manage if I went back to work and what to do if things deteriorated at home. We decided together in late September that it was time for me to go back to work.

I planned to go back on Monday 5 October. The Friday before, I went to meet Ronan Glynn and some of the key members of the team. I wanted to be briefed and ready for the following Monday. I remember looking at the numbers and listening carefully to Ronan Glynn's analysis. He was as worried as I was. He had chaired the NPHET weekly meeting earlier that week, but the deterioration in the disease as the week went on was accelerating, and was showing all the worrying early signs of exponential growth.

The five levels that we had devised to step down restrictions at the beginning of the summer were also those that would apply to any increase in restrictions. Level three was the next level in the national plan, but that weekend, none of us believed it could possibly be a sufficient pre-emptive and decisive step to halt the rapidly deteriorating situation. I spent that weekend phoning around the various members of the NPHET whose opinions I valued. Everybody was concerned. They all reported much greater concern about the data in the latter part of the week and what that signified. Again, no one believed that a level three response would be sufficient.

At this stage, I had never worked with Stephen Donnelly. My first contact with him had been as I was stepping away at the start of that summer. I sent him a text message on the Saturday, 3 October, before I was to return on the Monday to explain what I was hearing and seeing. That I was concerned with the numbers – by then we were at 400 cases a day – and that a NPHET meeting would take place on Sunday morning. I called the meeting for a Sunday because I wanted to ensure the minister would be in a position to advise cabinet of any change in advice at the next meeting, which would be on Tuesday (or sooner if possible) rather than putting it off until the following week.

The minister made contact with me on the Sunday morning and we had a conversation in which he asked to join the NPHET meeting. I explained my reasons for needing to have the meeting carried out without him being present – this being so that I could provide advice to him that I could trust and stand over. In the call, I was clear on my view that a county-level response would not be sufficient and that level three would not be sufficient. I was very clearly saying that the whole country needed to step up restriction levels, sooner rather than later. And that it had to be level four or five.

* * *

There was now a realistic prospect of having a vaccine in the coming months. I felt real hope that we could now see a pathway out of Covid. I believed that meant we had an additional obligation to redouble our efforts to protect people who were most vulnerable. Getting better control of transmission would protect them as they waited for a vaccine.

The NPHET met for some hours and came to a clear consensus. We talked it out through a series of questions which we considered one by one. I specifically asked for everyone to make a contribution to each question. I was always especially careful to do that when I believed we had an issue before us that could lead to significant new policy recommendations. That might not be the case at each NPHET meeting. But it was certainly the case on this occasion.

The first question was whether everyone shared the epidemiological assessment that we were facing a rapidly deteriorating position which was a significant and growing threat to public health and the operation of the health services. We did.

The second question was whether the measures that were now in place were sufficient to prevent further deterioration. Everyone agreed that they were not.

The next question was whether an escalation should apply to the whole country or whether we could maintain a response that simultaneously treated parts of the country differently. Again, there was consensus that the whole country should be as one in the application of restrictions.

The next question was whether a national application of a level three set of restrictions would be sufficient. Again there was consensus that this would not be sufficient.

We came to a consensus. Level five would afford us the best chance of getting control re-established. It had worked before. We had good reason to believe it would work again.

The advice was set out as usual in a letter on that Sunday afternoon. Prior to sending the letter to the minister, I arranged to have a teleconference briefing with Minister Donnelly in which I talked him through the details of the analysis and the recommendations. That was the first time I'd briefed him after a NPHET meeting, and I thought it important that he was the first one to hear this and that he heard it from me as chair of the NPHET.

It has been suggested that I should have spoken directly to the Taoiseach. But bypassing the minister and briefing the Taoiseach is something I had never done in my time as CMO. I only ever spoke to a given Taoiseach when they contacted me. It was particularly important that I respect Minister Donnelly's role, given that this was in effect our first time working together.

The letter was delivered to the minister, and copied in the usual manner to Elizabeth Canavan, assistant secretary in the Taoiseach's department, who I also spoke to by phone, to alert her to the outcome. It was for her to brief further as she saw fit within her department This would have been standard collegiate practice for me right the way through the pandemic.

A very short time after sending the letter, the news hit RTÉ.

It was said that somebody in the NPHET must have leaked it. Ronan Glynn and I were the only two NPHET members who had copies of the letter. And I know with cast-iron certainty that neither he nor I leaked. I have also known Liz Canavan for almost two decades and I know she did not leak it. Whoever did leak it knew there would be an enormous response in the media and among the public. I knew that too – and I knew that would prevent our advice being considered for what it was and acted upon as it should have been. And that is what played out.

There was a suggestion that I was the leak. That the government didn't like our advice, and so I decided to leak it to 'bounce' them into having to follow it. That was absurd. I would have known for sure that a leak would be counterproductive to any careful consideration of our advice, and all I was interested in was getting this advice heard. What I had hoped was that there would be confidential high-level discussions between senior officials, ministers and the Taoiseach. The seriousness of the issues at stake deserved that. Instead, someone saw fit to leak the letter, or its contents, which prevented any serious engagement with what the letter had actually recommended.

Whoever leaked that letter was absolutely determined that all attention be taken from what we were recommending. By then, public compliance was already reducing, and the controversy over this leak further eroded buy-in from the public, because now there was a sense of 'Them' and 'Us', a sense of division and mistrust.

Over the course of the pandemic, we did have a challenge with someone leaking confidential material from the NPHET. This was intended to, and did, cause great difficulty for us. It undermined the work we were all trying to do. It left us open to an accusation that we had an agenda beyond simply doing our jobs to the very best of our ability. I did take the opportunity to address the issue on several occasions in NPHET meetings. I made it clear that I regarded leaking as totally unprofessional. I used the strongest language I could find when I spoke about it. The last place I wanted to be as chair of the NPHET was commencing a meeting with a strongly worded rebuke and exhortation that I had to direct at the whole NPHET because of the unpatriotic, cowardly and unprofessional behaviour of one member.

* * *

The cabinet committee on Covid, which took place on Monday 5 October 2020, was difficult. I faced a lot of pressure and many difficult questions. The focus of the questions was not what the advice was saying, but how it had been formulated, shared and leaked. I stuck to my analysis and my advice: 'This is what the data is saying, this is what we need to do.' I was not about to change or soften the advice simply because it was not welcome. I believed it was the right advice and that it should have been acted upon. I knew in my heart and soul that we had not leaked this letter.

That evening I was at home with Emer and Clodagh, watching the *Claire Byrne Show*. Leo Varadkar, the Tánaiste, was on it. He talked about the members of the NPHET and how insulated we were from the effects of the advice we gave. He suggested that we were protected from the consequences of what we recommended because we had safe public sector salaries. That wasn't fair or true. We lived in the real world. We were impacted. Our families were impacted, financially and emotionally. Emer was slowly dying and would be cut off from all her friends and family in her last few months of life. We had family members who had businesses and relied on a fully functioning economy to make a living. The idea that we were somehow immune to the consequences of our advice was utterly unfair. He accused the NPHET of producing advice that wasn't thought through, which was absolutely not the case.

I remember how devastated Emer was. How conscious she was of how we had discussed the idea of me going back to work – the way we had weighed up consequences; what that decision meant for our family; and how driven it was by the sense both of us had that I could be of use to the country. There was very little I could say to console her. To her, this was a betrayal. 'How could he say that after all you've done? After we've made so many sacrifices? How can he possibly say that?' she asked. I had no real answer. Except that this was politics.

The next morning I got several calls from people in government suggesting they felt Varadkar had gone too far. It was clear to me that there was a fear that I might walk away from my job in response. In fact, hurt as I was, I had absolutely no intention of walking away. I was focused on the job and doing what needed to be done, and that had to take precedence over my personal feelings. Because we were clearly in trouble.

* * *

Over the course of the next two weeks, before our recommendations were finally accepted, we continued to monitor and report, and our advice remained unchanged. Two weeks went by in which disease transmission got much worse.

I was regularly asked in press conferences if I had spoken to Leo Varadkar, and he was also being asked publicly, had he spoken to me? Had he apologised? In fact he did ring me one evening, and the first thing he asked was 'How is Emer?', which I appreciated. We had discussed this before – Emer had been sick for the entire time that Leo Varadkar was Minister for Health, and he was a doctor – so I spoke a little about that with him. After that, he acknowledged that he had gone too far. He didn't apologise, and later, publicly, he said he didn't think he had anything to apologise for.

But he sent me a text a few days after the phone call, saying that it was good to have me back, and something along the lines of 'Let's do this.' He had completely changed his position on our recommendations.

* * *

The decision of the government to accept the NPHET advice was welcome. By then, we were reporting approximately 1200 cases a day. I feared that this meant the challenge of getting in control of the levels of transmission would be much greater now. The only change in the NPHET's recommendation was that the period of application of level five recommendations extended from four weeks from 4 October, to six weeks from 20 October.

These measures meant that there was a sharp reduction in incidence, hospitalisation, critical care admissions and mortality. In that time period, most of Europe continued on a path of increasing incidence, which led to levels of hospitalisation, ICU admission and mortality which were largely averted in Ireland. But as we approached the end of November and early December, the improvements we had seen in the preceding weeks started to reverse.

The NPHET held one of its longest meetings on 25 November to consider the question of advice to deal with the high and growing incidence of the infection and the risks that posed, especially to the vulnerable, as we approached the Christmas period. In the resultant letter, the NPHET clearly recommended that the hospitality sector remain closed over the following eight-week period.

My letter of 17 December 2020 noted:

The NPHET is especially concerned at how rapidly the case numbers have increased over recent days and notes that the epidemiological situation is considerably more concerning now than had been projected at the end of November. In particular, the timing of the current increase in cases is clearly related to the change in public health measures from the 4th December onwards. While it is difficult to accurately project the future trajectory of the disease at this stage, there are significant indications that we are now experiencing the early stages of a third wave of infection.

That Christmas saw a significant surge in infection brought about by high levels of socialisation. We saw a return to pre-pandemic levels of socialisation, which in my view was directly related to the failure to curb hospitality. That sent the wrong signal. 'If the pubs are open, how bad can this really be?' was what many people thought.

The NPHET met on a number of occasions over that period. We were profoundly concerned. The NPHET's recommendations were further added to by letters I wrote to the minister warning of the significant emerging dangers and the need for urgent action. This was made all the worse by the emergence over Christmas and into the new year of a new, more contagious Covid variant known as the Alpha variant.

Schools had to remain closed for a significant period even though we knew that the risks of transmission in that controlled environment were lower than in many others and that children were less vulnerable to the infection. School activity leads to very large-scale social mobilisation, which creates many additional opportunities for transmission. Furthermore, children share houses with adults and older people who are more vulnerable than the children themselves. For these times of such high transmission the NPHET believed it was necessary and proportionate to keep schools closed.

There were more than 1500 Covid deaths in January 2021. It was the single worst month for deaths over the entire course of the pandemic. This was at a time when we knew how to control the spread of the virus, but we failed to do so as a country. Many of the people who died were probably not far away from the point at which they could have been offered the protection of vaccination. I still cannot understand why pubs and restaurants were allowed to remain open over that Christmas despite the clear NPHET advice. It set the scene for a return to pre-pandemic levels of socialisation.

The timing of dominance of the new Alpha variant came too late for it to be the explanation for the case numbers we saw up to and over Christmas. Alpha made a bad situation much worse in January and catapulted Ireland to peak incidence in international terms. We had to revert to full implementation of level five measures, but did so much more slowly than was recommended by the NPHET in its correspondence in late 2020. The decisions made and not made regarding the advice from the NPHET, and also from me as CMO, as well as the signal that retaining hospitality gave, created the circumstances in which so many people died.

I cannot say that all of the deaths in January 2021 could have been prevented. But I think we should have prevented a lot more of them.

CHAPTER TWENTY-ONE
Emer's Last Days

BY A STRANGE, ALMOST eerie coincidence, Emer and her mother were admitted to Our Lady's Hospice and Care Services in Harold's Cross on the same day in late October 2021. Emer was admitted to the palliative care unit and Ita to the long-term care service. She had been transferred from St James's Hospital, where she had been ever since her stroke in mid-July. An astonishing coincidence. And a terribly sad one. But with some compensations.

The nursing staff were wonderfully kind, and since Emer and her beloved mother were effectively in the same place, they brought her over to visit her mum on a few occasions. These were the last three months of Emer's life. Her siblings weren't able to get to see their mother due to Covid restrictions, but Emer was. The effect of the stroke meant that Ita had limited awareness. That was very upsetting for Emer, but she knew that there was some protection in it for her mother.

* * *

During that spell in the hospice, Emer started to develop symptoms that suggested a spread of the disease to the base of her brain. There are 12 cranial nerves in that area that control functions such as eye movement, taste and smell, and some of these started to show problems. A CT scan showed that lesions in this area had grown to the point where there was a high risk that they might cause some serious problems. The question was what to do about that.

The usual answer was radiotherapy, but head and neck radiotherapy is a delicate business. Everything in the head and neck region is close to a vital structure, and there can be significant side effects.

Emer and I talked a great deal about the best thing to do. The team at St James's Hospital were helping us to explore the possibility of going ahead with radiotherapy, which would have involved Emer being admitted to Beaumont hospital. We were already at a point where the trips to St James's from the hospice were enormously depleting of Emer's energy and adding to her pain. At this stage she had stopped some of the chemotherapy drugs, because they were causing difficult side effects and it was obvious that in spite of the chemotherapy, the disease was still progressing. They were bringing no benefit.

After heart-breaking discussions, including with the palliative care team, we came to a decision. One Emer had already come to herself: she was not prepared to go through this for the limited benefit it would bring. She also wasn't prepared to risk losing her hair again. Indeed, if she had a complication while undergoing radiotherapy, she might have had to be admitted in Beaumont. In that event, given the deteriorating pattern of Covid, the probability was that Clodagh and Ronan wouldn't have been allowed to visit her.

That, for her, was the deciding factor. We began to make arrangements for Emer to be discharged from the hospice. That was what she wanted.

*   *   *

About a month before Christmas, Emer came home with a home care package in place and this was the only way it was possible. She was brought into the house on an ambulance trolley, and the ambulance personnel had to assist her into her chair in the kitchen. She wasn't able to walk. She wasn't able to use her right arm. She had a wheelchair but she couldn't propel it by herself. In fact she could do very little at all.

After a couple of weeks of being at home, Emer could walk unaided. That was such a wonderful improvement, something that meant so much to the children, who were able to see her almost as she had been. She was free of all the side effects of the drugs, and free of any of the side effects that might have arisen from radiotherapy. She was mentally alert and in really good form.

For me, this shows the benefit that can come from having a difficult conversation about the value of treatment and its goals. That conversation, with each other and with the medical team, led Emer to stop the active treatment with chemotherapy and radiotherapy. They were no longer helping and were leaving her with side effects. She was now free of those side effects and for a time she felt better and more able than she had done in a very long time. It was liberating.

Emer was home for about two months and lived in a way she hadn't done for quite a time before that. For the first time in a long time, it felt like she was getting better. Even though we all knew this wasn't so. We never quite said 'This is our last Christmas', but we both knew it. We steered away from using phrases like that, even though the heaviness was in both our hearts all the time.

On Christmas day I cooked, as I always did. It was just the four of us. Usually, Emer's parents and her sister Niamh and family would be there. I think that was the first time in 15 years that we were just four. It was our last Christmas together and it was lovely.

Emer went back into the hospice for the final time on 8 February 2021.

We did everything we could to keep Emer at home for as long as possible. When that was no longer possible, we managed to avoid an admission to St James's Hospital. Emer's wish was to die in the hospice. She was familiar with the environment and she had great faith and confidence in the staff.

* * *

Martha had died on 6 February 2019. She did well after initial treatment for cancer a number of years earlier but became ill again in late 2018. She arranged for all her family and friends to attend a screening of *Casablanca* in the Stella cinema in Rathmines. It was her way of saying goodbye. Emer last visited her two or three days before she died. It was a heart-breaking loss for Hugh and their children, Liam, John and Rachael, as well as the Ellison family. Emer was devastated by Martha's death. She was determined to stay in close touch with Martha's family, and especially Rachael, and she did that right up to the end.

Emer's last good day was Martha's two-year anniversary, 6 February. On that day, a neighbour had dropped in a belated Christmas present. Emer opened it and as she did, she and Clodagh made an 'unboxing video' for a bit of fun. In that video, the two of them are clowning and laughing. Later she had an anniversary Zoom call with Martha's sisters. At the end of that call, she had a dreadful headache. The headache continued into the next day. It was very positional, in that if she sat in a particular position, it would disappear, but if she moved, it came back instantly.

I didn't know what this was, but it was not good. Colin did a video consultation with Emer and changed some of her medication. By the following morning, the quality of Emer's voice had changed. I knew we were in trouble.

Colin came to the house and examined Emer and found that three if not four of the twelve cranial nerves were no longer functioning properly. I knew that if I called an ambulance and brought Emer into St James's Hospital she would be admitted onto the next available ward, where she would likely be unknown to the staff. Instead, we knew that the right step for Emer was to go back to the hospice. Clodagh and Ronan got to accompany her to the ambulance. No one said it, but we knew she wouldn't be coming home again.

I had worked until the Friday before that Monday admission. Because we lived so close, I was in and out three or four times a day. Clodagh was able to drive herself and Ronan, which meant he could study much of the time and pop in and out for short visits. The first few days after admission, Emer was engaged, talking to us and discussing the Leaving Certificate with Ronan. All she had wanted, since her diagnosis, was to be in our children's lives in a meaningful way. And she was. No matter how much her body was letting her down, mentally she was there for them as long as she could be. But after a week or so, she became increasingly confused and effective communication was no longer possible from Tuesday onwards.

I can replay those final days in my mind in great detail. On the day before Emer died, Clodagh and Ronan and I were with her for the whole day. Occasionally we went out to the rose garden on the grounds, a beautiful place and somewhere I had brought Emer many times on previous admissions, to get some space and some air, to walk and talk and make sure we were all ready. We knew by then beyond a shadow of doubt that the sooner Emer died the better it would be for her. We never wanted her to leave us, but we could see it was her time to go.

CHAPTER TWENTY-TWO

Emer's Funeral

EMER DIED AT 3.40 in the morning of Friday 19 February 2021. Clodagh, Ronan and I had been with her for most of the previous 48 hours. She had been unconscious since Tuesday evening and it was clear that she was dying; what wasn't clear was how long she might still last.

On Thursday night, Clodagh, Ronan and I went home to get some rest while Emer's sister Orla and brother Ronan sat with her. We considered the possibility that we might not be there if Emer died suddenly. We knew that was a risk, but we were conscious that this could go on for some days and we needed to ensure we were sleeping and eating as best we could.

We came home around half-eleven and went to bed. At about half-two I woke up and rang the ward. I spoke to one of the nurses, who said Emer seemed more or less as she had been when we left. That same nurse rang back just a few minutes later to say, prompted by my call, she had walked to Emer's room and had noticed a significant change.

We left almost immediately and drove the three kilometres to the hospice. Thanks to that compassionate nurse, we made it in time. Ronan, Emer's brother, stepped out to leave the four of us to be together for the last time. Emer was alive but her breathing had slowed substantially. The three of us gathered around her bed, held her hand and talked to her as she slipped away. Those final moments were very calm. The children were resolved and prepared. There was no sense of shock. This reminds me of these lines from 'Clearances' by Seamus Heaney:

Then she was dead,
The searching for a pulsebeat was abandoned.
And we all knew one thing by being there.
The space we stood around had been emptied
Into us to keep.

After Emer died, we stayed with her for another hour. We left at about six in the morning and drove home through quiet, empty roads. Around us, a few cars began to appear; the early risers starting to go about their day. Our lives had changed utterly while everyone else's simply carried on as normal. It felt strange that the world should continue as it had been, with Emer gone from us. But, of course, that is what the world does.

The three of us spent the day in the room we call the sunroom – a kind of conservatory where we have the piano and guitars. At the time, it had all the extra furniture crammed in that had to be taken from the TV room to create the downstairs bedroom for Emer. It wasn't that we talked all the time. It was more the desire to be with each other and support each other. We didn't wake anybody to share the news, but once it was properly daytime we began to let family and friends know.

At around midday I went to the funeral home – Massey's in Templeogue, where I met Mary Cunniffe. She was so caring, considerate and professional. It makes such a difference in a difficult moment like this to have someone like her. Emer's sister Orla came with me. I didn't bring the children. It's not that I thought it would be better not to have them there – I decided to let them stay at home. But I regret that. I found myself disconnected from them for that hour or so at a time when all I wanted was to be close to them. In that whole weekend, that's what I remember as being the most difficult.

Nobody could call to the house. We were in the midst of Covid restrictions, so not even Emer's family came. It was just the three of us, sitting quietly together. The death notice was published on RIP.ie that afternoon. And it was as though someone had plugged our phones into some kind of power source. They lit up. The volume of messages was unbelievable. We were overwhelmed, but also very comforted by the extent of sympathy.

The Taoiseach, Micheál Martin, released a statement in which he made warm references to Emer's work in the Department of Health in 2001. He had been the Minister for Health at the time. He recalled her work on the health strategy, Quality and Fairness, which was published in late 2001. He referenced the contribution she made and the experience of working with her. It meant so much to us all and especially to Emer's dad and her siblings to hear the Taoiseach's commendation of the professional contribution she had made.

The Taoiseach also rang me that day to express his condolences. We were in the car at the time, and when I told him this, he spoke directly to Clodagh and Ronan on speaker phone in a way that was warm and humane. I knew he had experienced grief himself, having tragically lost two children, and I felt he understood something of what we were feeling. I also received a call from President Higgins, which meant a great deal to us all.

Emer's death was on the news that evening, and in the newspapers on the following day. I still have all those weekend papers. One day I plan to put them all into a scrapbook, so the children can have a record of the wonderful things written about Emer.

*   *   *

On Saturday morning, we had to go to Mount Jerome cemetery to pick a grave. It was a miserable rainy February morning, the kind that makes you want to stay in bed. And so wet that we were advised to wear wellington boots.

It sounds like the most awful task – choosing a grave for your wife and mother – but in fact, it turned out to be strangely enjoyable.

Emer had wanted to be buried here. This was one of the conversations she and I had – we had used the Think Ahead materials from the Irish Hospice Foundation to structure our talk. It is a beautiful graveyard, very close to where we live and even closer to Lower Kimmage Road where her dad grew up. He is buried there too now, as are Emer's grandparents.

While the street entrance to the graveyard and the hospice are not immediately adjacent to one another, their grounds mostly adjoin and are separated only by a high stone wall. Emer's last room in the hospice was close to the dividing wall between the hospice and the cemetery. In a way that seemed fitting.

We spent about an hour, me, Ronan and Clodagh, walking around, guided by Alan Massey. He was a wonderful guide, and told us all about the history of the graveyard, the different customs over the years, and the differences between a reconditioned grave and a 'new' grave. Emer had specified a re-conditioned grave – the least expensive – but in the end that was the one wish of hers we didn't respect. We chose a grave to the side of the stone church, near a row of yew trees and surrounded by beautiful old historic headstones.

In the afternoon, we spent some time finalising the words we would say on the day. Clodagh and Ronan had decided that they wanted to contribute to the eulogy, so they went upstairs together and wrote their own pieces.

* * *

On the Sunday, Emer was laid out at the funeral home, and both families paid staggered visits at 15-minute intervals. Clodagh, Ronan and I went first. After we left, Emer's dad, Frank, and her siblings came, one by one, with their individual families, followed by my family.

Afterwards, they all came by our house in their separate groups. We stood on the front doorstep while they stood in the driveway in the freezing cold. This was the first time Clodagh and Ronan had physically seen many of their cousins for quite some time. We had been restricted, more or less, since the previous autumn. It was the only way to do this, given the circumstances. They couldn't come in. They couldn't come to the funeral. They couldn't even give us a hug. That was very hard. But we knew we needed to maintain complete compliance. There was a genuine risk that someone somewhere might try to catch us doing something outside the restrictions and record it, and we knew we couldn't have Emer's funeral hijacked by that.

Deciding who could attend the funeral was easier than I might have expected, given the size of the family. We could only have ten people, which meant just the most immediate family: Emer's dad, her three siblings, my parents, myself, Ronan, Clodagh and the priest.

Beyond this immediate circle, everyone else – in-laws, cousins, friends and so on – stayed at home and watched online. It is not the same as being present, but it was better than nothing – when it worked. The funeral was broadcast live, but was so heavily subscribed that the feed crashed several times. We didn't know that at the time, but we heard many people couldn't get to see it as a result. I guess that was a sign of the scale of the outpouring of love and emotion for Emer.

For months afterwards, people I didn't know would meet me and say 'I tuned into your wife's funeral . . .' That was such a lovely thing to hear.

* * *

Emer was in Massey's funeral home in Templeogue village on the funeral morning, Monday 22 February. As we were about to go in, I heard someone call my name. I turned to see Hugh Mulcahy, Martha's husband. He was there with his daughter, Rachael, who was only 13 when she lost Martha in 2019. And here they were to support us. Then I realised that Martha's sisters were standing across the street. Suddenly, I felt over-whelmed. I was caught completely by surprise.

It is in moments like that that my emotions get the better of me. When I'm not ready. And there were many of those moments over that day. I think of the line in Seamus Heaney's 'Postscript' where, perhaps by different emotions, he is over-taken suddenly: 'And catch the heart off guard and blow it open.' That was me at that moment – caught off guard, my heart blown open.

I realised that some of our closest friends were also standing on the other side of the road. It was very difficult that I couldn't go to greet them. I could only wave from a distance and make hand gestures to say 'thank you'; communicating across the street via body language, with buses driving up and down between us. That was strange and unsatisfactory and goes against every human instinct – to be close to people in times of trouble. But it was also amazing that so many people had made the effort to be there for us in the only way they could.

The route the funeral cortège took from Templeogue village was towards Bushy Park, then left to travel along the perimeter wall of Terenure College towards the church. I was driving my own car behind Emer. Ronan was in the front seat with me and Clodagh was in the back. As we turned left at Terenure College, there were all of Ronan's sixth-year classmates, in full uniforms, together with teachers, standing socially distant one from the other, lining both sides of the road as a full guard of honour.

Father Éanna, the principal of Terenure College, had kindly rung to tell us this would happen, but even so, we were over-whelmed by the sheer scale of it. It was a highly emotional moment. Many of these young men had shaved or extravagantly dyed their hair as a dedication to Emer to raise funds for the Cancer Society and for Our Lady's Hospice. Emer knew about it and was aware to the point when around €30,000 had been raised. Eventually they raised close to €80,000.

We turned left again into the last stretch towards the church, and there too were people on both sides of the road who we hadn't known were coming. We could only take in little bits of it. I am still emotional when I recall the moment. I saw friends and relatives and kind people from so many parts of our lives. In the churchyard were two uniformed military personnel – the President and the Taoiseach had both sent their aides-de-camp to formally express their condolences, which was so appreciated by all of us.

And then, inside the large church – where Emer and I were married, where she was baptised and made her first communion and confirmation – it was just that small number from our two families.

* * *

The priest who said the funeral mass was Father John Browne, a County Down hurling man. He is a Spiritan priest who lives in Kimmage Manor, where he originally trained to be a priest, after a lifetime of missionary work all over the world. Emer met him in St James's Hospital where he was introduced to her by another chaplain, the irrepressible Sister Joyce. She was a ray of sunshine lighting up the rooms and corridors of St James's Hospital. We got to know her well over many years and her visits to Emer were like a medication – always a boost.

Emer liked both Father John and Sister Joyce from the moment she met them. So it was natural that she wanted Father John to say her funeral mass. The parish priest at St Pius X in Terenure was very understanding and was agreeable to Father John saying the funeral mass. Father John brought a daffodil with him and spoke of it as a symbol. He didn't know until later that Emer loved daffodils. She loved spring and Easter and the hope that time of the year brings. That daffodil travelled on the coffin with her, and went into the grave with her.

We had put a lot of effort into the music for Emer's funeral. We couldn't have a live performance in the church, so Emer's sister Niamh and her colleagues in the wonderful St Pius X Folk Group created a CD with all the individual pieces to be played.

Clodagh, Ronan and I all play music. Clodagh has completed all her piano grades and is very proficient. Ronan plays guitar and I play guitar. The three of us had recorded a Glen Hansard song, 'Falling Slowly', a favourite of Emer's, in the days before she died. The three pieces were brought together to make it sound like we had performed together. Emer got to hear it in the hospice before she died.

We also played a beautiful song performed by Lisa Hannigan. It is called 'A Prayer for the Dying', and I believe she wrote it about a close friend's mother. Lisa and I have a mutual friend,

Una Molloy. She knew I was a big fan of Lisa Hannigan's and how particularly poignant I found that song in the context of Emer's illness. Lisa recorded a video of her singing that song for us and Una sent it to me on the Sunday before Emer died. We listened to it together in her room in the hospice, just the two of us. It was a special and tearful moment.

Finally, we played another of Emer's (and Ita's) favourite songs, 'Bright Blue Rose', written by Jimmy McCarthy. Again thanks to Una, McCarthy had heard that Emer loved this song, and he sent us a recording of himself singing it, which I think is the very best version of all its recordings.

We had all this wonderful music that was special to us. Clodagh, Ronan and I delivered the eulogy together. We stood side by side at the altar as we delivered our eulogy to an almost-empty church, but it didn't feel like that. We were speaking to each other, to our family, in a way that was lovely, peaceful and intimate.

*   *   *

It was a bitterly cold afternoon. The burial was attended only by those of us who had been in the church. Then we drove out of the graveyard and went home. Alone. That was when the effect of Covid restrictions seemed most cruel. I worried about the children coming back to the empty house. I felt there might be a sense of flatness after a funeral; of 'now what?' as you realise the busyness of those first days is over, and you are left with the awful realisation of loss.

Knowing that, we asked family and friends to call to the doorstep over the course of the afternoon. They came at planned intervals and stood in the front garden driveway while we stood at our front door. Barbara considerately brought squares of pizza. Later, Ronan's pals arrived, complete with dyed or shaved heads after their fundraiser. I heated the pizza and they stood in a circle, socially distanced, for half an hour eating warm pizza. As a group of 18-year-old lads, they were happy. And Ronan was among them, laughing too. After they left, Clodagh's friends came by. It was getting dark at this point and again they sat in a large circle with their coats on, chatting. Neither of them had really seen their friends for months, and I could hear lots of laughing. Emer would have loved that. I was happy to hear that they could still laugh even in the middle of their profound grief.

When we closed the door that evening, I remember feeling the emptiness. We had been carried through the day by many kindnesses, by the funeral and all that had to be done during it, and by seeing people physically even if we couldn't hug and embrace them. Now it was the three of us. We had a video call with Martha's family and, finally, a video call with my five sisters.

We had got through the day and the funeral. One step at a time.

*   *   *

In the days after the funeral, we had to find things to do, ways to cope and ways to move forward. I didn't go straight back to work but I kept in touch with the office. As a family we had been through so many gradual adjustments at home over a long period of time with Emer's illness. There was a good deal to do in sorting out the house. We had had a lot of adaptations as Emer became more unwell, and we wanted to restore the rooms to what they had been. First, there was a lot of equipment that we no longer needed, including a hospital bed.

For a few days, Clodagh would go into the now unused room and lie on that hospital bed. That was hard to see. I didn't want to rush her, but neither did I think it would be helpful for us to let the room become a shrine. Clodagh and I talked about this, and about returning the large volume of specialised equipment that we had accumulated – walkers, a wheelchair, the various pieces of equipment that Emer had needed.

We gathered everything together into the now unused TV room. It was poignant to see the trappings of Emer's illness in one place. Once everything was taken away, it was equally poignant to look at the empty room. So one day, when Ronan and Clodagh were still in bed, I slipped out and bought a new TV, put the couch back in and got the room set up as it had originally been. By the time they came downstairs, the work was all done, and the room was again a place to relax and switch off.

I felt that if I went back to work with practical tasks not done there was a risk they wouldn't get done. So I was determined to keep tackling the chores. I also needed to keep busy, and tidying and sorting out rooms, cupboards and drawers was work that was time-consuming but not taxing. Exactly what I needed.

We needed to decide what to do with Emer's personal possessions; her clothes and so on. We discussed all this; Clodagh wanted to keep just her jewellery and a small number of things. There was a particular shirt Emer used to wear that we turned into a toy bear. I gave some precious items to people who were close to Emer, and the rest went to charity. A goldsmith, Eva Dorney, melted Emer's wedding band with mine, and made them into one new ring that I now wear on my right hand.

*   *   *

I stayed off work until after Clodagh and Ronan had returned to school and college. About three weeks after Emer died,

Covid guidelines enabled Leaving Certificate students to return to school, and Ronan felt he was ready. Clodagh was in first year of university studying physiotherapy, so she continued to attend lectures online for a few more weeks.

The big focus, for the three of us, was Ronan's Leaving Certificate. That is what Emer had wanted, and that was what we concentrated on. I spent a lot of time cooking. Because I had time, I put effort into preparing good meals for the three of us and that gave a structure to my day.

After dinner on weekdays, Clodagh and I would walk with Ronan the short distance to Terenure College, where he went to after-school study. Then she and I would continue for a walk in Bushy Park. At the time, her relationship with her boyfriend was coming to an end. He was a lovely fellow, a real source of support for her during Emer's illness and a great person for her to talk to. We walked, and talked a lot about that. And how she was adjusting to Emer's death. That was what I was really most concerned about. I was worried about how this break-up might impact her grief. I definitely worried – and I still do – that I can't be a father and a mother to her and to Ronan. I'm trying to be as much as I can, while being mindful that I can never fill the gap Emer left.

I'm conscious of that now and was very conscious of it at the time. I asked for advice from my sisters. I continued to encourage Clodagh to express herself. In fact, Clodagh herself taught me the lesson I needed most, by saying to me, 'Dad, I don't need you to fix this, I just need you to listen!' That was very wise of her. It didn't come as naturally to me as it would have to Emer. But it was a very valuable lesson and one I was grateful for. I'm not sure I have any advice beyond this for anyone else who finds themselves in a similar situation, but that is what I try to do and I believe it has been very helpful.

CHAPTER TWENTY-THREE

Time To Go

I WENT BACK TO work on 19 April, exactly two months after Emer died. By then the epidemiological situation with Covid was getting much better. It was clear that there was room to accelerate the relaxation of restrictions. There was understandable caution, given the experiences we had had, but the NPHET advised strongly on the need to move on as quickly as possible from the restrictions.

Many people had already been vaccinated, starting with those in high-risk groups. Vaccination was being rolled out on a risk-prioritisation basis and the capacity to vaccinate was growing. I hadn't been vaccinated myself at that point, but an appointment wasn't far off. The delivery of the vaccination programme was a major logistical undertaking for the HSE and one it managed very well.

I think there could have been greater understanding in the upper ranks of the HSE of the need for the logistics to follow the science and data on both safety and efficacy of vaccines. Very few of them, however, had been through the experience of swine flu and narcolepsy. A vaccine programme for a new vaccine needs to be flexible enough to respond to changing evidence about efficacy, effectiveness and immunogenicity (the capacity to provoke an immune response). It simply must be very responsive to any safety signals that arise, even when there is a risk that these signals might be false alarms. While that will sometimes create headaches for the logisticians, it cannot be otherwise.

One example of this followed a decision to temporarily halt use of the AstraZeneca vaccine based on safety considerations. Ronan Glynn was acting for me during my absence after Emer's death. He was decisively taking the only responsible action he could following advice he had received from the National Immunisation Advisory Committee (NIAC), yet there was open criticism of this decision by some who ought to have known better. In making that decision and in following through on it, he was adhering to principles that underpinned our approach to the pandemic response, including a commitment to communicate early and often, to be transparent, to act on the evidence available to us at a point in time, and to be prepared to be dynamic and change course if that was required.

The vast majority of people wished to be vaccinated as quickly as possible, but it took time to get the HSE programme up to peak capacity. The minister and government felt there was room for improvement. And the public was impatient. That was a good problem to have – other countries faced indifference and scepticism. It is very clear that trust in vaccines was maintained at high levels. I am clear that the reason for this was that the public believed in and trusted the advice that was given on the vaccine. So did I.

That advice came from NIAC, which was chaired by Professor Karina Butler, a highly respected paediatrician. NIAC is a body of experts that operates under the aegis of the Royal College of Physicians and that has provided independent and trusted advice and guidance on immunisation policy and practice for almost three decades. Their advice on Covid vaccines changed as the evidence changed. It could not be otherwise.

A new vaccine programme has to have agility and adaptability to allow changes to be made as the data and evidence demands. That is especially true when it comes to safety-related data. It was clear to me that the willingness of NIAC to change their advice when data and evidence suggested they should was a key reason that the public maintained such a high level of trust in the vaccine programme. Trust is key to vaccine uptake. We have seen many examples of that over the years.

The HSE ran a very effective vaccination programme. It drew in significant voluntary support and was a clear example of the whole country pulling together. It was a time of hope and optimism as more and more people received their first dose. I remember queuing up for my vaccine in the Aviva Stadium. There was a constant flow of people in and out. The queue never stood still. The whole system ran smoothly and quickly. A well-oiled machine.

Over the course of that summer into early autumn of 2021, we achieved a higher vaccine uptake than almost any other country in Europe and there is no doubt that social incentives were a significant part in driving that and protecting the population.

We were conscious from the outset, in all our conversations around vaccines, of the potential for anti-vaccination senti-ment. We have had examples of this over several decades. There were claims about the diphtheria, tetanus, pertussis (DTP) vaccine in the 1970s. In the 1990s there were the claims made by the discredited and disgraced Andrew Wakefield in relation to the MMR vaccine and a link to autism. In the 2000s, it was HPV vaccine complications that included chronic fatigue and other alleged syndromes.

Anti-vaccination groups are better funded and organised, and more coherent and proactive in their communications, than ever before. We have had to develop major campaigns to promote the benefits and to refute the alleged complications with HPV. Through the efforts of Laura Brennan and others we have recovered ground that was lost, and that is good news for the prevention of cervical cancer. There is a small anti-vaccination community in Ireland which includes people who are dedicated to spreading misinformation and fear. The evidence of Covid and other vaccination programmes is that it has not had as significant an impact on vaccine uptake in this country as it has elsewhere.

There is no room for complacency, however. The anti-vaccination cohort is growing. Furthermore, over the course of the pandemic we saw the emergence of all manner of vague pseudo-scientific and conspiracy theories spreading through social media and via key influencers. It seems to me the challenge of tackling disinformation and misinformation is growing and will continue to do so. We need to get better at pre-empting and responding to that.

The expert staff of the Department of Health's communications office were monitoring social media and were able to judge the extent to which any of this was gaining traction. We incorporated this knowledge into our communications as much as we could. For a large part of 2021, our press conferences and regular communications included experts on vaccination. We made sure we had good, credible, authoritative people to be part of those press briefings.

When a question around vaccination safety arises, I treat it as a serious question. I know that many people, particularly parents and pregnant women, have a genuine and rational need for information and to make informed choices. It was our duty to make the information as clear as possible for these concerned people. They may have read something in a newspaper or on social media that raised questions for them, so it is right that they have those questions answered, whether by their GP or through a well-organised information campaign.

Not every question that arose during the pandemic needed to be addressed. Our press team would have received invitations along the lines of 'Why won't you come and debate such-and-such a person?' The media might think they're offering a balanced perspective, but the risk is that you elevate somebody without credibility to a position where they appear to be taken seriously. If, for example, Andrew Wakefield and I appeared on a radio programme to discuss the MMR vaccine, that is not balance. You must avoid the risk of enabling them to have equal weighting and giving them credibility.

There was a small number of medical doctors and scientists in Ireland who expressed anti-vaccination views or played down the impact of Covid. They risked damage to public health which, as far as I am concerned, raises questions about their ethical standards. While I fully accept the need for free speech and for legitimate questions to be raised, their actions gave legitimacy to disinformation and misinformation. There was a spectrum of these doctors. Some had genuine but false views and sought opportunities to put forward these views. Some were in positions of influence and used those positions to spread false information, doubt and fear.

And then there were others who were simply contrarians, who saw opportunities to promote themselves. Among these were a few who specialised in radio and television programmes and writing columns in newspapers. It didn't really matter what our view was, theirs was always contrary. Very few of them made clear how their expertise was relevant to the points they were making. Some of them shamelessly gave opinions on their chosen subjects with no more expertise than anyone else. I think there is something unethical about that.

A medical practitioner is not a layperson. The position of privilege that comes with being a medical practitioner comes with a solemn duty and responsibility to first do no harm. That should extend to all our activities as doctors, in my view. A media 'debate' between doctors can lead to people becoming genuinely confused. And confusion often means that people may not take action, i.e. not get vaccinated.

A medical practitioner must understand the limits of their own particular expertise and the impact of their public communications on a population. I think it would be very useful for the Medical Council in its own reflections on the pandemic to consider more specific guidance on public communication by medical practitioners on matters of public health, particularly during times of declared public health emergencies such as a pandemic.

*　*　*

After Emer died and as 2021 progressed, I began to think about what next. I felt myself at something of a crossroads personally as well as professionally. I needed to think holistically about my life. Clodagh and Ronan had finished school and had started college. After a year and a half of almost non-stop Covid crises, Ireland was getting to a much better situation. It had been a very intense time for me professionally and personally. I was pretty tired.

When I thought about what life might be like after moving on as a CMO, I imagined that international public health might interest me. I thought about working with the WHO or going into academia. Nothing was clear, but I had a sense of a wider world and a need to find new challenges for my own progression and development. I was also mindful, as I have said earlier, that I didn't think having the same CMO for 24 years or more (I was appointed at 41) was good for the role.

I talked to a couple of close friends and, over the course of the summer of 2021 decided that it was the right time for me start planning to move on. In August 2021 I spoke to Martin Fraser, secretary general to both the Department of the Taoiseach and the government, who I knew well. I also spoke to Robert Watt, secretary general of the Department of Health.

It wasn't that I knew exactly what I wanted to do or where I wanted to go. It was more a sense that I needed to create space and give myself time to look at opportunities. As part of this, I arranged to go to Spain for a complete break in the first week in October. I hadn't been abroad for about five years at that stage, since the last trip Emer and I had taken with Clodagh and Ronan.

I went on my own as Clodagh and Ronan were busy with college. That took a little bit of courage, I admit. I was going to the same place we had visited many times as a family, Sunset Beach Club in Benalmádena. That meant I was very familiar with it, but there were also a lot of memories there. But I felt it was important to confront it. I knew it would give me a chance to think.

As it turned out, by then cases were rising quickly. That was the beginning of a wave of Covid through the end of 2021 and into early 2022.

* * *

The entire winter from that point on was dominated by the demands of the disease. The Omicron variant emerged in late 2021. At first the hope was that it was less severe, but there was no certainty about that. What was clear at the outset was that it was more transmissible. Greater transmission means a bigger public health issue, even if the severity is no worse for the individual, because it leads to many more infected people.

By late 2021, the public appetite for our messages about new variants and new measures was greatly reduced. So too was our own appetite for issuing such messages! More restrictions was the worst possible news to be giving and we took no pleasure in imparting it. I was determined that if we got evidence that this was indeed less severe, we would remove the restrictions as quickly as we could. We held a NPHET meeting during the first week in January 2022. At that point there was hard evidence that this variant was much less impactful at the population level and especially in a population as highly vaccinated as Ireland's.

The NPHET therefore agreed that we should advise the early removal of restrictions. We recommended that the government remove all the restrictions in two steps, one at the beginning of January and one at the end of January.

By February 2022 we made a clear statement, reflected in the advice of the time to government, that the emergency phase of Covid was now over. We were moving into a different phase with different requirements. That is when we, as the NPHET, made the recommendation to bring the NPHET process to an end.

The pandemic had been lengthy, the issues complex, the effects on people through deaths, illness and wider social and economic impacts had accumulated and we all became weary and impatient for it all to end. But I was always clear that there could be no change in the seriousness of our obligation to provide the best possible impartial and good faith analysis and advice to government and to the public. At times, that involved difficult conversations. But I believed in what I was doing. I believed in the people I had supporting me. And I believed in the necessity to speak truth to power and not to be afraid to do so. When it was most necessary, it was also most difficult.

The ending of the NPHET signalled the 'end' of Covid in many ways, although I certainly don't believe Covid is fully behind us. We will also have to deal with long Covid. More research, better definition and service development and long-term services will be required. In particular, it will be important to define the most relevant disciplines when it comes to leadership responsibility for patients with long Covid. The emergence and scale of long Covid is another reminder of the importance of Covid vaccination and the need to achieve much higher uptake of the vaccine among the groups in the population to whom it is offered.

* * *

As my mind was turning to new opportunities, I was acutely conscious of the high likelihood that we will see another pandemic in the next decade or two – soon enough that we should be concerned, yet far away enough to see most of us who were part of the Covid response retired. I was therefore very minded to ensure that I could find opportunities to apply learnings I had developed over the course of the pandemic.

One specific question is that of human resource capacity and how central it is to our capacity to respond to any public health emergency. What challenged us in Covid was *scale* rather than *complexity* per se of a number of specific tasks. Many relatively simple tasks were required at unprecedented scale and took longer than was ideal to mobilise and to put in place. Examples are contact tracing, administration of vaccine, carrying out swabbing and implementing basic infection prevention and control guidance in vulnerable settings – and there are many more.

The execution of many of these tasks during the pandemic required the redeployment of professionals who need not have been redeployed had we been better prepared. This carried an enormous opportunity cost in terms of service provision. Services had to close or be curtailed as a result of this. We should not need highly trained nurses to vaccinate and emergency medical technicians to swab, for example. We cannot in future rely on deploying expensive and highly trained health-care staff (and closing or limiting their services) in order to support basic public health tasks that are essential to health protection.

If we are to have resilience for future pandemics and public health emergencies, we need to bring together a wide range of tasks and knowledge of basic 'public health literacy' and competence into a module of basic training which should be common to all health professionals, so that we diffuse this basic knowledge through our healthcare system. This will need to be developed through a common curriculum, an accreditation and certification system, and be reflected in the scope of prac-tice descriptions of a variety of professionals in our system of professional regulation.

But if we are to have real resilience in our future emergency response systems, we need to create a new type of capacity at scale and well connected into local communities of people who have knowledge and skills that can be mobilised without pulling highly trained health professionals from their core duties. Keeping health professionals working in the health system is an essential part of protecting public health.

We therefore need a new workforce in an informal and voluntary capacity that is mobilised as and when needed, to work in a system of delivery and clinical governance that is reflective of such a role. In my view, being able to mobilise voluntary community-based capacity will be an important determinant of future social resilience in the face of pandemics and other major public health emergencies. Perhaps people could be paid when the role is activated. But they would be ready and waiting to deploy their skills, like a lifeboat crew or a civil defence.

Conceptually, I see this as sitting between public health literacy and formal healthcare education of health professionals.

I think of the census enumerator capacity and how it springs from nowhere to an instant capacity in every community: enumerators are paid when they work but not otherwise. There are many ways it could operate. As a voluntary activity, as a civic duty, as an incentive/qualification towards more formal higher-level qualifications. And there are national social or sporting and other organisations who could collaborate. Many issues will no doubt arise with staff, capacity, planning, professional regulation, etc. One of my personal ambitions is to create an opportunity to work on this and to find the necessary funding to make it a reality in the years ahead.

* * *

On a personal level, although my mind had been turning towards the idea of leaving from August, the disease prevented me from taking any real steps in that regard through the whole of that winter. Now that we were beginning to see light at the end of the tunnel, I felt this was my window.

Emer's first anniversary was coming up. We were planning a mass for our families and friends because the funeral had been so restricted. I decided I would get through that, and then I would take some time off to make the necessary arrangements to move on.

CHAPTER TWENTY-FOUR
My Secondment

BY THE TIME OF the final NPHET meeting on 17 February 2022, I had come closer to understanding what I wanted to do next in my career. It was two days before Emer's first anniversary.

The pandemic had really brought home to me how precarious and unsustainable modern living had become. It showed how urgently we need to find innovative and sustainable responses for the future of humankind, the planet and the fragile ecosystems on which we depend. As a public health doctor, I felt motivated to explore these issues and to contribute to understanding and responding to these realities with which we must contend.

I therefore felt compelled to go further upstream for a second time in my career, just as I had when I moved from clinical medicine to public health almost 30 years before.

My interest in health and wellbeing as resources for happiness and fulfilment, as well as economic and social productivity, was as passionate as ever. My wish was, therefore, to strengthen the knowledge and practice of public health leadership in this regard and forge stronger national links with the EU and the WHO. I wanted to spend more time than I could in my role as CMO thinking about health and wellbeing in a wider context of ongoing global issues including climate change, energy and water distribution, biodiversity, conflict and migration.

I believed that there was an opportunity in the context of this wider view of health and wellbeing to develop and to deepen ties between academic, health service and government stakeholders in one national collaboration to make progress on these goals. I believed that the international response to the pandemic in both the WHO and the EU would bring new funding, learning and leadership opportunities. A unified national collaboration would provide us with the best means of deriving benefit for Ireland from these opportunities.

It was my view that the academic sector was the right place to seek to build such a national collaboration and to build a future-oriented leadership that would apply the lessons of the pandemic. That was the reason I wanted to take my journey upstream to the academic sector.

A secondment would provide a means of leaving my role as CMO but remaining on the same terms and conditions and continuing to work on public health within the public service and in a manner I believed would benefit the country.

I talked through all of this with both Martin Fraser and Robert Watt. Through those conversations, I was assured that there would be support for me to be seconded, assuming that the work was relevant, and all the parties could agree. I would remain working on improving public health and applying Covid lessons in the academic sector. This was in a context where Ireland needs to significantly invest in developing capacity for a much stronger public health system for the future.

This is a road that had been travelled by people at secretary general level. Formal specific secondment guidance for someone at my level of seniority or for secondment to academia from the civil service did not exist. Later, there was a lot of discourse in the media about the rules of secondment. Secondment is a beneficial tool in the public service that allows people to share and grow their expertise in different areas, fields and sometimes international agencies. But the reality was there were no specific guidelines for this type of move. Such rules as there were covered a move from one government department to another (and at more junior grades), not the move from a government department into the public service.

While I was not a secretary general, both Martin and Robert believed and advised me that the process used in those cases would be the right precedent for my proposal, although, given that I was not a secretary general, it would not require a formal government decision. Martin advised me to seek further advice from one of the recent secondees at secretary general level, which I duly did. I had all the support I needed from both Martin and Robert. I had no reason to believe it would be anything other than a straightforward matter to progress. I took some much-needed annual leave to work on the details of a proposal.

* * *

At the start of my annual leave on Monday 21 February, I had a preliminary short meeting with UCD to determine their interest in my proposal to be seconded to develop a public health leadership programme, and to create a full professor post to lead it. On 22 February, I met with the Provost of TCD and outlined my ideas. Both universities expressed initial interest in my proposal. It was clear that neither would be in a position to fund the role – that would not be required if a secondment was approved. I didn't approach other universities as I didn't wish to be based outside Dublin and away from Clodagh and Ronan so soon after Emer had died.

I now had a plan: go back, talk to the necessary people in the department, and put together a clear description of what

I would do, what Trinity or UCD would do, to make clear what we were all agreeing to. Trinity acted faster and therefore became the focus.

A letter was issued by the Department of Health on 16 March 2022 and signed by Trinity, laying it all out clearly. My new role at Trinity was to be Professor of Public Health Strategy and Leadership. The Department's intention was to commit €2 million collaborative research funding a year, to be administered via the Health Research Board and made available competitively to all universities. The letter provided for further details to be worked out between the Department and Trinity.

To me, this felt like a perfectly reasonable proposition. I was going to continue to make my expertise, such as it was, available to the public service. This is where my interests have always lain. I have never sought to enrich myself. In my profession, I could have gone down a completely different route from a specialisation point of view, if I had wished to earn more money. I didn't. I was making a decent salary that I was perfectly happy with. What was important to me was the value of the work, by which I mean the value it delivered to public health and wellbeing in Ireland. This is what has driven me from the earliest stage of my career.

Robert Watt signed a letter to me to say that this was a secondment; I needed that documentation in place to make sure that I was protected and wasn't giving away my rights and pension entitlements, which is, I think, reasonable. I signed a letter to say I wouldn't at any point look to go back and be CMO again – even if the Trinity position didn't work out as intended. I was under no obligation or pressure to make such a commitment, but I wanted to enable the Department to set about filling the job permanently out of respect for the role I had held for so long.

* * *

Robert Watt had been at the Department of Health about a year at this point, having previously been secretary general of the Department of Public Expenditure and Reform (DPER) for many years. He and I had a perfectly straightforward relationship, and discussed all of this in a straightforward way.

For the avoidance of all doubt, I know that Robert was genuinely trying to be helpful. At my level of seniority, it was technically a matter for him, rather than the minister, to approve. What was different about this was the pandemic. I now had a profile, albeit one I did not seek, which had to be factored into thinking about who needed to approve or be aware of this. I was informed and believed that all the necessary briefings of people who needed to be aware, particularly the minister, had taken place.

From my point of view, we were where we needed to be: the Department was agreeable. Trinity was agreeable. I was agreeable. Everything was in place.

Until it wasn't.

By now it was mid-March. For their part, Trinity had to bring the appointment through their own system of approval. That process was due to run until lunchtime on Saturday 26 March. While I could not control it completely, I wanted this news to be as tightly managed as possible out of respect for the process in Trinity. I wanted to make sure they had the space to approve, or not, in their own way without speculation in the media.

On the Wednesday before the Saturday deadline, I received an email from an *Irish Times* journalist: 'I hear you're leaving your job; can you confirm this is true?' Followed by three or four more questions. I ignored it, and no story appeared in the *Irish Times*. That told me that he had heard rumours but didn't have any corroboration.

However, early on Friday afternoon the same journalist was back again. 'I'm going to run the following story unless you get back to me to tell me it is not true.' The cat was clearly out of the bag. Somebody somewhere had given him the information – I had my suspicions but I didn't know anything for sure – and now he had the bones of the story and was going to run with it. A statement was prepared, approved and issued in the name of the Department and the minister. But it turned out the minister was less conversant with the details than I had believed.

The announcement was made on the Friday afternoon, and got quite a lot of attention in the media. That surprised me. Taoiseach Micheál Martin made a public statement and reflected positively on my time as CMO and the service I had given, which was pleasant.

At some point about a week later, the Department's press office received questions from RTÉ and in answering those, the word 'secondment' was used. Then somebody within the government said, 'I didn't know it was secondment,' and this began to be portrayed as something that was being done in secret; something that was inappropriate.

All of a sudden, all sorts of important people were able to say, 'I didn't know about that.' The inadequate communication meant that the news breached a political golden rule – the 'No Surprises' rule – and caught people on the hop.

* * *

The following Monday evening I spoke with the minister by telephone about new advice that I had received from NIAC. During that call we spoke at some length about my proposed move. I explained that this was a secondment, that I was not improving my terms and conditions, and would continue to work on public health matters of relevance to the country. I talked about a big opportunity that was then on the horizon, around new European health funding. A new agency was being created by the EU – the European Health Emergency Response Agency – of which I was the Irish board member. I could see the scale of the EU ambition to grow and align budgets, including research budgets, for public health emergencies and related funding.

I felt this was a great opportunity for Ireland if we could unite universities, the HSE and the Department of Health to work on joint proposals and projects. I explained that I hoped to work on such a collaboration as part of my Trinity role. I wanted to see what we could do as one nation, competing for a very significant increase in inward investment; and how we might use that to build capacities around research and response.

Certainly I had no sense during the conversation that he was unhappy with my move or that he had any unanswered questions about it. The following day, he appeared on *Morning Ireland*, was asked about it and gave a very positive response.

But others weren't so inclined. Michael McGrath, then Minister for Public Expenditure and Reform, was asked for his views, and he said he knew nothing about it, that his department hadn't sanctioned the move. In the space of a few hours, my departure turned into what looked like an evolving story – one where new facts appeared to be coming out.

On the Thursday morning of that week I was invited to attend an Oireachtas Committee hearing on a matter of public health. The meeting was conducted in private session. I was asked about the Trinity appointment. I explained my position. But unfortunately, none of this took place in public.

The following morning, I was driving Clodagh to college when the radio news came on. The Taoiseach was in Helsinki, and as I listened, he began to say – in response to a question from a journalist – something about not having enough information about my Trinity move, and wanting the whole thing to be paused pending a full report. I turned the radio down immediately. I didn't want Clodagh to listen to this. In any case, I didn't need to hear any more. I had heard enough, and I knew what it meant. I knew that the move couldn't now happen. The Taoiseach had said he wanted this paused, which would mean months of questions, and weighing up of answers, before any kind of conclusion could be reached. All the ingredients of a long-running affair were in place.

I went home after dropping Clodagh. Martin Fraser rang me. The first thing he said was, 'I don't know what to say to you . . .' That said it all, really, about where we now were. He also told me to expect a call from the Taoiseach, because he had been told this would happen – that Micheál Martin wanted to talk through what he had been quoted as saying in Helsinki, on the basis that this had been misreported to an extent. No phone call came, and I haven't heard from him since.

I knew I had a big decision to make, and I wanted to make it properly. In fact, the decision was clear. I knew I was not going to hang around for this drama to play out. I particularly felt a responsibility not to have Trinity dragged into it. There was really only one decision for me to make. I sat with it for a little while, and spoke to a couple of close confidants, but I felt was that there was only one right thing to do. I would announce my intention to resign from my job.

I was very disappointed, but I was also reasonably accepting. These things can happen. Political controversies can occur out of all sorts of things, and often they have limited – if any – relationship to the facts. This was one such.

There were mistakes made, clearly, in the way all this was handled, but there was nothing inappropriate in what was being proposed. People might say, 'Oh, but now they're going to be paying for two CMOs,' but the truth is, we need to radically increase our capacity for senior-level thinking in public

health terms. A lot had already been said publicly and politically about the need to do this, and there was general
agreement across government that we needed to put more
money into research and public health understanding. This
was a chance to make good on that.

When the report was eventually published in March 2023,
the pointed nature of media queries that I received made it
very clear that selected material from the report was being
leaked in advance of publication and 'spun' to create damage
for me and to unfairly shift responsibility to me for what had
happened.

I could not ignore this. I immediately took the opportunity
to write to the minister, as the commissioner of the report, to
express my concern. I believed he, as commissioner, had a duty
of care to me and to the truth. I was genuinely at a loss to
understand how after more than twenty years of loyal public
service to the highest professional standards, circumstances such
as these arose in which a proposal which I developed in good
faith and which had only progressed when it was clear that it
had the prior knowledge and support of Secretaries General
Watt and Fraser resulted in such unfair and unbalanced
portrayal of me in the media.

I had taken the decision to resign from the Department
in part to limit distraction to the minister, his government
colleagues and senior officials arising from the fall-out of how
my proposed secondment was handled by those I relied on. In
the same spirit, I refrained from public comment at the time
beyond my initial statement welcoming the publication of the
report.

A conclusion in the report stated that I was 'exclus-
ively personally involved in the negotiation of research funding
linked to my possible secondment'. No facts were set out in
the report to support this conclusion. Although I am not clear

if the reviewer believed that I was or not, the media were quoting this conclusion in such way as to suggest that I was negotiating funding levels for health research with the universities. That interpretation of the conclusion in the report is completely false and without foundation. There was no discussion or 'negotiation' at any stage with either of the universities on the level of research funding. Had anyone sought to establish the facts, I am certain that each university would have confirmed that I did not discuss or negotiate research funding with them. Robert also knows that this claim is false. The only discussion to which I was a party that encompassed research funding was with him.

It is gratifying that almost everyone thinks it would have been a good idea. I welcome the public statements from the minister, the Taoiseach and the Tánaiste that everyone acted in good faith. They clearly do not believe that I was involved in such an inappropriate and conflicted manner. If the minister and DPER had been appropriately informed, I am sure that the proposal would have proceeded.

*   *   *

In all of this, the question arises – do I believe that I received fair treatment in the overall handling of my proposed secondment, subsequent report and related commentary? No, I don't.

The clear and true facts are: I came up with a good idea. I proposed it first of all to Martin and Robert. I had their informed support. There was a failure to inform and clear it with the relevant people. The responsibility to inform the minister, DPER and the Taoiseach was not mine. When the idea ran aground, I took the decision to quickly move forward in a different direction by resigning. That was my decision and I believe it was the correct one.

CHAPTER TWENTY-FIVE

Leaving

On 9 April 2022, I announced that I would resign as CMO on 1 July. This left plenty of time for the process of finding my replacement. After the considerable disappointment of the handling of the Trinity opportunity, I decided it would be best to seek to develop a portfolio of activities that would be of interest to me rather than one single new job.

In May and early June, it looked as though Covid case numbers were going up again. At that stage, the CMO job still hadn't been advertised. I still had weekly meetings with the minister to brief him on Covid. On one occasion, after I had finished briefing him about the rising case numbers, he said if I decided I wanted to stay past July, I would have his full support. I thanked him, but I was not for turning at that point.

He wasn't the only one to suggest something similar. In fact, at one stage it was suggested to me that I had an obligation to stay until there was a new person in the role. Someone from HR said that as I hadn't yet given formal notification of resignation, my notice period was not sufficient. They implied that I would have to stay past 1 July. My response was, 'If you want to operate on the basis that you are the only person in the country who doesn't know that I'm going on the first of July, then by all means we can have that conversation.' I didn't hear any more about it.

It was time to go, and I was ready.

I felt too young to retire and do nothing. I passionately believed there was much more I could contribute. I have never pursued career goals based on money and I don't have complex financial arrangements. With two children in college, I wasn't in a position to retire.

Now that I had made my announcement, I found myself reflecting on my 14 years as CMO. I suppose a certain amount of reflection is to be expected. I had time to run my mind over the time I spent in the role, the issues I worked on and the people I met along the way. I felt the privilege of having served in the role. Over the course of this book, I have written about some of the bigger and more high-profile issues I was involved with. But there were many more that deserve mention.

Healthy Ireland, an ambitious cross-government policy, was published and approved by government in 2013. I was proud to have championed the case for its development with ministers James Reilly, Frances Fitzgerald, Róisín Shortall and Kathleen Lynch after they took office in 2011. Its premise is that wider integrated actions across society and government are needed to address health and wellbeing and, in particular, health inequalities. We received committed support from the WHO's Regional Director for the European Region Zsuzsanna Jakab, and her successor in that role, Hans Kluge, as well as Professor Sir Michael Marmot from the Institute for Health Equity in London. Their support was critical to building the necessary political support we needed. One of the more innovative aspects of the policy was the creation of the Healthy Ireland Fund, which provides funding for initiatives in other sectors which are intended to have a positive health impact. I think it was a missed opportunity that proposals we developed in the

Department of Health to have the dividend from minimum unit pricing for alcohol and from the tax on sugar-sweetened drinks redirected to grow that fund further and to enhance its impact were not supported by the Department of Finance.

Although I was involved in all manner of issues, one of the hardest, and certainly the most long-drawn-out, was alcohol. The work began in 2009 with the appointment of the National Substance Misuse Strategy Group, which I chaired, to tackle public health harm caused by alcohol. It published its report in 2012. The group included representation from the Alcohol and Beverage Federation of Ireland (ABFI) and Drinkaware, which is funded by the alcohol industry. While I was supportive of their inclusion, I had come to a different view by the time they tabled their dissenting minority reports.

What made the process additionally difficult was the resistance from other sectors of government. Opposition to proposals as they progressed through the various stages of the decision-making process were more sectoral than political in origin. With the notable exception of Frances Fitzgerald, the Minister for Children from 2011, the Minister for Health was often a lone voice at cabinet in promoting the measures we proposed. It was through the persistence of successive Ministers for Health (Harney, Reilly, Varadkar, Harris and, especially, Minster of State Marcella Corcoran Kennedy) that we got to the point of enacting legislation – the ground-breaking Public Health (Alcohol) Act 2018 (a law to limit the harm to public health of alcohol consumption) – while preventing it being so watered down as to be meaningless. One person whose role was pivotal was Alex White. He took over from Róisín Shortall as Minister of State for Health in 2012 and continued to support the proposed legislation when he was later promoted to a full cabinet position as Minister for Communications.

The final Act provides for: minimum unit pricing; health labelling of alcohol products; the regulation of advertising, sponsorship and marketing of alcohol; separation of alcohol products in mixed trading outlets; and the regulation of the sale and supply of alcohol in certain circumstances. Many of its provisions were subject to extraordinarily long commencement periods and requirements. Some are not fully implemented, with opposition coming from interests not only in Ireland but among EU member states. While most of these regulations have been signed into law, some as late as May 2023, it seems certain that national and international vested interests will continue to resist their effective implementation.

Ireland developed quite a reputation for tobacco legislation. I was privileged to lead the team responsible for standardised packaging and the transposition of the EU directive on tobacco products, which was advanced significantly by Ireland's presidency of the EU in 2013. Legislation was also introduced to prohibit smoking in cars where children are present. We also developed the policy and advanced legislation to license the sale of tobacco products, including cigarettes, and although the progress on this was impeded by the pandemic, it is now at an advanced stage of development. We must reflect, however, that while progress has been made, one in five over 15s are daily smokers in Ireland.

Over the course of my time as CMO, policies were developed and approved by government to address obesity, including a tax on sugar-sweetened drinks and the National Physical Activity Plan, which was jointly developed with the Department of Tourism, Culture, Arts, Gaeltacht, Sport and Media. We also introduced developed policies on the prevention of sexually transmitted infection and to prevent skin cancer, which included legislation to regulate the use of sunbeds.

I was also responsible for public health and health service policy development and the establishment of related public health programmes to monitor, prevent, manage and mitigate impacts related to major health risks, including infective, environmental, patient safety, behavioural, chemical and radiological threats.

A specific threat to highlight in this regard is antimicrobial resistance (AMR), which is concerned with bacteria that are resistant to antibiotics (often colloquially called 'superbugs'). The Chief Veterinary Officer, Dr Martin Blake, of the Department of Agriculture and I led a One Health response to AMR by co-leading a national stakeholder group to develop two successive three-year action plans, a central component of which was the creation of a single One Health AMR surveillance report with data relevant to antibiotic use and infections relating to both humans and animals. One Health is an integrated, unifying approach to balance and optimise the health of people, animals and the environment.

Another example related to health system strengthening is patient safety. Triggered by an investigation of a series of neonatal deaths in one maternity unit, a National Patient Safety Office was established in my division to drive clinical effectiveness into health service operation through new national clinical practice guidelines (many related to infection prevention and control of healthcare-associated infection) and national clinical audits and to implement a National Patient Safety Surveillance System to enable early identification of health system failures. It also led to the National Care Experience Survey, which measures, analyses and reports on patient and user experience of health service use.

The work on these issues helped to build the capacity for evidence synthesis that now exists in the Health Information and Quality Authority. It is an essential function which grew during the pandemic and now supports clinical guideline development; the National Screening Committee established following the Scally Report on CervicalCheck, and NIAC.

We also advised and supported policy development work right across the Department of Health in relation to all aspects of the health system, including Sláintecare, the government's national health system reform plan; the National Cancer Strategy, published in 2016, following on from the 2006 National Strategy, the development of which I was closely involved with; and policy in relation to chronic diseases and rare diseases.

The work was always varied and interesting. Its reward came from the sense of privilege I felt to have a role that could influence important issues that impacted the public and that were meaningful in everyday life. I loved the variety, and every day felt like a new and refreshing challenge. It might not have had the immediate gratification of a clinical role, but after 14 years in the job, I was able to look back with pride and satisfaction on the work we had done, the contribution I made and the impact it had.

I have received awards, which honestly surprised me, from many organisations, mostly as a result of my role in Covid, most notably the Freedom of Dublin, which I accepted on behalf of the health system and of the NPHET and my core team. I didn't ever feel I was 'owed' anything additional for the work I did as CMO and during the pandemic. For me, the opportunity to do the job I did was its own reward. Some may take issue with the advice or recommendations I gave, but no one can take issue with the fact that I gave my job as CMO the very best that I could. The last thing I was ever going to do was to change my advice because it suited someone politically for me to do so. I don't believe that is what anyone would expect of me, or wish from me. I am proud to stand on the record of my leadership of the public health actions undertaken by the Irish people during the pandemic.

*   *   *

The CMO job continued to be busy into the summer, but I avoided getting drawn into any new projects. I needed to preserve some mental energy to figure out what I was going to do next. I felt I was leaving a world I knew extremely well, and going into a world that was very new. I was going to have to consider and create opportunities for myself. UCD appointed me as an Adjunct Full Professor of Public Health in the College of Health and Agricultural Sciences in UCD in July 2022. UCD took a strong leadership step in creating this college, which supports the One Health vision, in 2015.

I have had a series of engagements with the WHO in relation to One Health and I hope to be able to create an effective collaboration on this agenda between UCD and WHO. I am also working with the WHO country office in Baku, Azerbaijan on strengthening their public health system. The work with WHO is focused on the essential elements of public health and is both invigorating and interesting.

In September 2022, I was appointed to the board of the Irish Hospice Foundation. The foundation is an advocacy and fundraising organisation whose purpose is to raise awareness and improve the experiences of people around death, and support that through providing services such as nurses for night care and the materials that it creates.

My interest in the areas of bereavement and death didn't just stem from Emer's illness. As I have written earlier, Emer completed a needs assessment for palliative care. Her research brought her to look more closely at the operation of specialist palliative care services and into questions around location of death and how those varied across populations. She looked at audits of the effectiveness and performance of palliative care services in other countries and the value of extending palliative approaches to care to other settings including hospitals and homes. She and I talked a lot about all of this while she was working on the thesis. We both felt concerned that so many people in Ireland die in acute hospitals, which are challenging environments both for those who are dying and for their loved ones.

Then it came to pass that Emer ended up using palliative care services, and so we saw them from a new perspective. Emer used the Think Ahead guide to help us through some of the more difficult, but necessary, conversations. Through that process, we learned at first hand how vital it is to be guided through these with simple, usable materials designed to allow the hard questions to be addressed more easily, and to record the answers one by one at a pace that is comfortable and comforting.

*   *   *

When I have to explain the differences between clinical medicine and public health medicine or the factors that influence our health and wellbeing and the complex way in which they are rooted in our environment and how our societies and economies function, I use the analogy of a river rising in the hills. It flows downhill, through countryside, villages and towns. It is joined by other tributaries. It grows as it goes. People have to cross it, use it to travel, to power mills and to water fields. In bad weather the river can flood, burst its banks and wash homes and villages away. While the river brings life, people do fall in or get washed away. Some of these people drown.

As a doctor in clinical services, you try as best you can to save individual people who have fallen into the river. As a public health doctor, however, I think differently. I think of how fast it flows, its tributaries, how wide it is and how long its course is. I try to understand why people are falling into the river in the first instance and how to prevent them from doing so.

I've given a lifetime of professional commitment to public health. It is what I am passionate about. It motivates me. It has always held my interest and always will. The issues I was involved with during my years as CMO have a unifying theme: making health and wellbeing central to our definition of living well and making it central to everything we do and invest in. That was the central purpose of the Healthy Ireland framework, published in 2013. It sought to create a single public policy focus on health and wellbeing, a prerequisite to successfully addressing the many challenges facing society.

I see health and wellbeing as essential assets for happiness, fulfilment and personal growth as well as vital resources for sustainable economic and social functioning and productivity for individuals and society as a whole. I left clinical medicine to pursue a career in public health at a relatively young age. Although I had completed my training as a general practitioner I was much more interested in wider questions of policy, of health inequalities, of disease patterns and other factors which I was less able to influence as a GP. I went upstream.

This river analogy works well for Covid-19. Here was a new disease, much more transmissible than influenza and more severe. There were no drugs to treat it. No vaccines to prevent it. And no natural immunity from previous viral variants. It was a river flood surging downstream and threatening major impacts on health all over the world.

Focusing on downstream issues alone would not protect people sufficiently. We had to try to reduce the risk of getting the illness, to reduce the size of the inevitable flood and to buy time for science to develop vaccines and treatments. All we could control, or influence, was the speed at which this disease was transmitted. If we could influence human behaviour.

The patterns of Covid-19 have highlighted inequalities and vulnerabilities among individuals and populations. Each of these is a tributary of the river into which people can and do fall. And the downstream consequences of Covid are almost infinite, reaching into almost all sectors of society, the health system, education, trade, service, tourism and industry. The Covid-19 pandemic has exploited upstream weaknesses in planning and in operational responses to public health emergencies all over the world. It has revealed and exploited gaps in societal security and resilience in the face of major emergencies. It has made clear that many assumptions and implicit wisdoms on which societies, economies and healthcare systems are based are flawed or false and entirely unsustainable.

My experience of Covid has reinforced my fundamental interest for my own professional future in looking at ways to influence the health and wellbeing of the population, starting with how we frame and value health and wellbeing as societies. I am interested in finding new and better ways to unscramble these issues and make them accessible so we can talk about them more and understand the actions we need to take. We need to see health and wellbeing as essential resources for economic and social productivity, personal fulfilment, and happiness. In order to do this, I believe we need to make a vital switch to holistically measure success and failure rather than rely on a narrow monetary definition of what constitutes success.

For decades, gross domestic product (GDP) has been the most used indicator to measure economic growth. It is a narrow measure derived from a model of economic theory that fails utterly to appreciate the complexity of unbridled economic forces and the devastation that the pursuit of GDP-only growth has wreaked on the planet through policies that steal from the future of the many to bankroll the present of the few. The narrow focus on GDP fails to value the wellbeing of individuals and societies in modern society. GDP only measures economic output, not the quality of life. It does not consider the distribution of wealth, environmental impact or social inequality. It does not capture the informal economy and non-market activities such as household work, volunteering, and caring for children and elderly family members. These are crucial to the effective functioning of our society. What would our lives be without them? The contribution of these activities to wellbeing and societal development is often overlooked and undervalued by traditional economists and policy-makers.

The emphasis on economic growth and GDP can lead policy-makers and politicians to prioritise short-term gains over long-term sustainability and wellbeing. This is harming our environment and exacerbating social inequality. It leads us to categorise spending on education, healthcare and infrastructure, which are essential for long-term societal development, as costs for our present rather than investments for our future.

It can be said that some aspects of wellbeing – happiness, mental health, social cohesion – are intangible and difficult to measure. But they are critical for a comprehensive understanding of wellbeing. Recently, there has been a growing recognition of the limitations of GDP as a measure of wellbeing. Alternative measures have been developed to provide a more comprehensive understanding of societal wellbeing.

The UN's Sustainable Development Goals (SDGs), adopted in 2015, are a universal call to action to end poverty, protect the planet and ensure that all people enjoy peace and prosperity. The SDGs comprise 17 goals and 169 targets aimed at tackling a range of global challenges, including poverty, hunger, gender inequality, climate change and environmental degradation. While they are global in focus, they provide a much more holistic means for every country of examining its actions in the present and plans for the future. The SDGs are essential because they provide a framework for global co-operation and action towards achieving a sustainable future for all. The SDGs require collaboration and partnerships across all sectors of society, including governments, civil society, the private sector and individuals.

Perhaps five or ten years ago, the call to action was just a set of goals and aspirations. Increasingly, however, some countries have made a conscious decision to move in this direction. They act as exemplars for other countries. Politicians and policy-makers, therefore, have more examples that help to show how this can be achieved with political will and appropriate policy choices. And, perhaps even more important, citizens can be empowered to make choices in how they live, consume and vote by being inspired by the sense of possibility that the practical examples of other countries offer.

Some of these countries have come together in a Wellbeing Economy Governments partnership (WEGo). This is a collaboration of national and regional governments interested in sharing expertise and transferable policy practices to advance their shared ambition of building wellbeing economies. WEGo currently comprises six national governments: Scotland, New Zealand, Iceland, Wales, Finland and Canada.

Why not Ireland?

CHAPTER TWENTY-SIX
Difficult Conversations

THERE IS NO WAY to confront the realities of an illness like multiple myeloma without a series of extremely painful conversations. From the time Emer was diagnosed, she and I talked about the diagnosis, its implications, the treatment and likely effects. We also talked about what would need to happen for our family, and particularly for the children, as the illness progressed.

These were difficult conversations, but they were important and valuable. Conversations about illness and death are not only helpful to the person who is going to die, they can also make things easier for those they love and will leave behind. Having wishes clearly communicated and written down provides comfort for those who remain; a feeling that they are carrying out their loved one's wishes.

Families and friends are left with a burden of grief following the death of someone close. But they are also left with practical issues that arise and decisions that have to be made, of which they may have little, if any, experience. For example, a grieving and bereaved person may have to decide what to do with items that had value during a person's lifetime, but have no natural home or value to anyone else after their death.

They may feel unable to make a decision, or guilty if they give things away.

Conversations may come more easily to some people than others. I think people can be supported and helped with them. We may need to find ways to be given 'permission' to have difficult conversations. Sometimes we might feel that by talking about what is to happen when someone dies, we somehow hasten it or even appear to be alright with it. Unless given permission to talk about death, many of us will avoid those conversations.

* * *

Emer and I first drew up our wills when she was admitted to the hospice for the first time in 2017. We didn't know then how much longer Emer was going to live, although she lived for nearly four more years. The children were still under the age of 18 so we had to talk about the possibility of guardianship if something also happened to me. I wanted to make sure I understood exactly what Emer's wishes would be in that circumstance.

Thinking about those possibilities was hard and those were very difficult conversations. That was probably the first time we spoke acceptingly and purposefully about what might happen after Emer died. We had had plenty of conversations about her prognosis, her treatment, and we had talked through all the bad news as it came; but that was the first time we discussed in practical detail what she wanted for Clodagh and Ronan and me after her death.

I know it wasn't the first time she thought about these things, however. She left a number of letters, written to me, the children, her parents and siblings. She kept these in a specific place that I knew of, and would very frequently remind me not to forget about them. She wrote these letters at different points in time, because what she needed to say changed as the children got older and as her illness progressed.

The first letter to me was written in the year after her diagnosis, and it is clear from reading it that she was living with an ever-present fear of early death and the impact of that on the children. That first letter shows me how important it was for her to write down what her wishes were, what her hopes and aspirations were for them.

During one of her hospice admissions, the Irish Hospice Foundation's Think Ahead planning materials were made available to us and we used them to put a shape on our conversation and her wishes. The planning materials have been developed and tested over a number of years and are an extremely practical and comprehensive guide for having such difficult conversations.

The Think Ahead guide takes you into practicalities at a very detailed level, and stresses the importance of writing down key information, such as bank account numbers, and wishes around funeral arrangements, for example what you want to wear when you are being laid out – and even your Netflix password.

Knowing that you don't have to cover everything in one go helps to make such a conversation less daunting. It allows you to make a start and see how that feels as you ease your way into it all. Emer and I found there was value in being able to talk for maybe 20 minutes, write down a certain amount, and then just put it away for another day. She was very good at saying, 'I feel good that we have done that and that is enough for today.' We got through it in that way; bit by bit.

Emer was able to express all her views and answer any questions around the funeral and those arrangements. This was a good thing for her. It brought her a sense of relief, of things being squared off and resolved. Even though it was very difficult to talk about a world that carries on after her death. It was very painful; I can see that clearly in what Emer wrote in her letters. She didn't want to die. She expressed that view even a couple of days before she died, in one of our last conversations.

Talking with healthcare professionals about future medical care options can improve quality of life and can help with mood and mental health. It can enable patients to have the benefit of palliative care at an earlier stage, as Emer did. We invest increasing proportions of healthcare expenditure to provide expensive treatments to people in very advanced stages of illness and well into their final year of life while knowing it may have limited benefit.

Often there has not been an honest conversation that gives a patient the clear understanding that some of these treatments are likely to be of limited or no benefit. The evidence is that many patients will opt for less aggressive care at the end of life if their doctors help them to understand that it is of limited value. Emer experienced the liberation of that in her final two months of life when her quality of life improved as a result.

In this context, the Think Ahead Planning Pack encompasses a tool to develop an advanced healthcare directive (AHD). An AHD allows future treatment choices to be made known well in advance of when they might be needed, in the event that a person no longer has the capacity to make choices. It also allows a person to be designated to speak for someone if they no longer have the capacity to make their own decisions. An AHD can now have a legal status, which will require healthcare professionals to take it into account in their decision-making about care.

The majority of us will never need an AHD and it will be voluntary for people to complete one. But I would strongly advise it, because if it is needed it is of immense practical value and comfort to patients and families. Ideally, every hospital or nursing home admission would routinely encourage the completion of an AHD, which will help to normalise their use. However, research shows that currently many patients do not share their thoughts and feelings about death with their doctor, and most conversations about death that do take place are not initiated by doctors. Emer and I benefited from these conversations and from thinking ahead and prompting the right conversations with her medical team.

There is widespread understanding of the value of completing a will. Similar understanding should attach to the value of having power of attorney arrangements in place, and a completed Think Ahead pack, including an AHD. The more we can normalise these in the same way as we have writing a will, the better and easier these conversations will be. It is important not to wait until the point of admission to hospital or until some serious illness arises.

Doctors have many opportunities to initiate these important conversations. Early conversations during outpatient clinics and in-patient admissions can give patients control over their remaining time. If it becomes clear that treatment is no longer effective, conversations should take place about symptom management, preferred place of death, and required support. These conversations need to be given adequate time. In the context of pressured health service delivery, that can be difficult. Some doctors find these conversations emotionally difficult. But they should be happening more routinely.

Unfortunately, these conversations are often put off until they cannot be avoided and then they are held in crisis situations, in emergency settings, with clinicians who have not had time to build a relationship with the patient.

* * *

One of the most difficult conversations Emer and I had was around what might happen for me in the future. Specifically other relationships. She brought it up maybe half a dozen times over the course of her illness, particularly towards the end. Understandably, that was something she found especially hard. She would get very upset during these conversations.

Nothing confirmed to Emer the reality that she would die more clearly than talking about me in a new relationship. I tried to deflect and change the subject and tell her that we didn't need to talk about it. But she wanted to hear me say that I was open to the idea of another relationship, and for me to know that she hoped for this for me. We knew how much we loved each other. I would tell her nothing could change that. But she insisted that I had to let her express herself. She also talked about it in the letters she wrote to me. She wanted to talk about her hopes that I would meet somebody and enjoy a future with someone else.

I am now in a lovely relationship with Ciara Cronin. Emer helped me to see myself moving on after her death by being clear in her wishes for me, and now that I am with Ciara, I feel grateful to Emer. Telling Clodagh and Ronan was always going to be a sensitive moment, but because Emer had written down her thoughts, and they had read what she had written, I was able to talk to them quite easily and openly in a way that I don't think would have been possible if this hadn't been discussed between Emer and me first.

Telling Emer's family was also an important step. I told Orla first, and as soon as I said it, her response was 'Emer spoke about this. It is what she wanted for you; to meet somebody.' All over again, I was grateful that we had talked about so much, and that Emer had said this to Orla.

Ciara is very much a part of our lives. She, Clodagh and Ronan are very fond of each other. I know that Emer and Ciara would have liked each other. There is a source of comfort in that for me.

I say the same thing to myself as I always say to Clodagh and Ronan – we're not trying to get over Emer's death. That is absolutely not our objective. We're trying to figure out how to live our lives in spite of the fact that she has died and that we have experienced a profound loss that we're not ever going to get over.

Emer will always be part of our lives. The love Emer and I had for each other will never die. And to ensure that, our natural conversation in the house brings her in and out. When Ciara is around there is no feeling of self-consciousness about talking about and making references to Emer in our conversation. Clodagh, Ronan and I are comfortable with Emer being spoken of in that natural way. I don't see that changing and we don't want it to change. It is a balance we try to get right and I think we have managed to do so.

As a final reflection on this, a few months after Emer died, Ronan and Clodagh in particular started to beg me for us to get a dog. I was open to the idea, if uncertain about the practical implications. We talked about the pluses and minuses and how we would share the duties. I instinctively felt it was important to make haste slowly on it. And then Ciara came into our lives, and her dog, Milis, fulfils that 'doggy desire' role for Ronan and Clodagh in a way that is very sweet. We often collect Milis from Ciara, for example if she is away, or very busy, and Milis fits into the house as 'our' dog for a few days. The best of both worlds!

*　*　*

I've always been something of an optimist. I've faced a lot of personal and professional challenges that maybe should have made me wonder about the basis for my optimism. In spite of those challenges I am mindful of all the wonderful things in my life. I had a wonderful marriage for over 25 years, filled with happiness, to Emer, whom I knew and loved since I was a teenager. We were blessed with two wonderful children, Clodagh and Ronan, with whom I have a very close, loving and supportive relationship. Emer prepared them so well for life as well as for her death. I am grateful that her love and support still guides us and it is the reason we've been able to find a way of living healthily and happily after her death.

I am very aware, however, that throughout our lives there will be moments when we will feel the loss and grief every bit as much as we felt it in those early days after she died. I feel sad for my children when I think about the special times in their lives that they have yet to experience and will not be able to share with their mother. I worry about her absence as a source of love and support at the times when Clodagh and Ronan face their own personal challenges. My parents are still alive and I'm very glad that they were there throughout my life. Emer had that experience also with her parents, who were a source of love, presence and support all through her life. Clodagh and Ronan had to lose their mother at the age of 20 and 18. I feel sad and powerless when I think about that. No matter what I do, it won't be enough.

Clodagh and Ronan are at university and forging their own paths in life. I love that they still live with me and I am very much a part of their lives. I love when their friends call to our house – belting out songs with Clodagh on piano or Ronan on guitar. It makes me recall how much Emer wanted our house to feel like a welcoming place for their friends and how much she enjoyed the sound of a gang of the children's pals. She always wanted Clodagh and Ronan to grow up feeling those are important values for their own lives.

I'm enjoying the first year following my departure as Chief Medical Officer. I have no regrets about my decision to leave. What I particularly enjoy is the feeling that I don't quite know what the next number of years will bring professionally. That is a new feeling for me. It has opened many opportunities for me and I hope opportunities will continue to come my way. It allows me to choose the things I want to be involved in.

I have managed to find a balance between work and personal life that always eluded me in my former role. I have more time for my children and my personal health, and I have time to spend with Ciara, who is a source of joy and optimism and hope for the future.

Emer's courage and open-hearted approach to life and death inspires me and guides me every day. I am a lucky man indeed to carry her love in my heart. She made everything possible.

Acknowledgments

I could not have achieved anything alone. Throughout my life and my career, I have been privileged and humbled by the support and encouragement I have had from so many people.

Emer was the most important person in my life. She believed in me, she loved me and she shared my life from when I took my first steps into adulthood until the day she died in 2021. She gave me reason and purpose. She celebrated my successes, comforted me in my failures and above all was always there. She is still there in my heart and I carry her memory and live by her values as best I can.

Emer and I had two wonderful children, Clodagh and Ronan, who have grown into wonderful young adults full of life. I am grateful for them and I thank them for everything they are and how much a part of their lives they have enabled me to be. They have encouraged me and supported me, especially in the time since Emer died. We are very close and I am thankful for that every day.

I have also had unwavering belief from my parents, Liam and Brigid, and my five sisters. We are in close touch. My parents made many sacrifices in their lives so that my sisters and I could have opportunities that my parents couldn't have. They instilled values and principles in us which have informed and influenced me, perhaps more than they realise, in the choices I have made in my own life and career. I am grateful for that.

My sisters are Therese Maguire (Kilkenny), married to Mark and mother of Cathal and Eoin; Aileen (Grappenhall, Cheshire), partner of Gwendy Gibson; Breda Considine (Limerick), married to Tom and mother of Brian, Emma, Aisling, Rory and Ava; Sinead Rhatigan (Kilkenny), married to Niall and mother of Sarah and Aoife; and Aoife Stoddart (Dublin), married to Colin and mother of Ailsa, Aidan and Caoimhe.

A few years ago, prior to the pandemic, my sisters and I started a WhatsApp group voice call every Saturday morning – usually as I walk around Bushy Park. It has been a real help to me to have access to their wisdom, advice and humour on a weekly basis. I want them to know how important this was for me. They all contributed thoughts on this book project, but I especially acknowledge Aileen for reading and re-reading drafts with patience and application.

Emer came from a wonderful family and a home that I was first welcomed into on St Patrick's Day 1987. Ita gave me tea and chicken sandwiches, served on bone china plates; I was on to a good thing! From that point on, Emer's parents, Frank and Ita, and her siblings, Orla, married to Philip and mother of Matthew and Stephen; Ronan, married to Niamh and father of Shauna, Donal and Aidan; and Niamh, married to John O'Brien and mother of Conor, Sean and Ciara, have been part of my life. When we were in college, Ita used to send me a bag of groceries every so often, which Emer would carry on her bike. It was the 1980s and I think Ita worried about this poor young lad from Limerick living in dingy flats in Rathmines and Ranelagh!

Emer's family are very close and they live nearby. Whether it was babysitting, Ballybunion or Sunday afternoons at Nana's, the Feely family closeness, warmth, love and support was always evident. I am privileged to have married into such a wonderful family and to still have them in my life. It was so hard and so unfair on them to lose Emer. She relied on all their love and support and I have no doubt it helped her in every aspect of the challenges of her illness to have it and to have the comfort of such deep and loving family relationships.

The other Feely family members won't mind me singling Orla out for special mention. She has been a friend and support to me for many years, but especially in the years of Emer's illness and after she died. Her intellect, wisdom and generosity of spirit was always available and was invaluable to me in recent years. She gave generously of her time in reading drafts of this book, in spite of the challenge of Frank's illness and death and the competition for the presidency of UCD.

Emer and I had wonderful friends. Martha was very close and for many years provided Emer with practical help and psychological support until her untimely death in 2019. Emer missed her greatly.

My dear friend Colin Doherty was at times involved in Emer's care. But he was also a wonderful friend and supporter. He was always there since I first met him in 1985. Understanding. Interested. Compassionate. Loyal. I think most people go through life without finding such true friends. I often think I have taken much more than I have given from that friendship. He was another to take on the challenge of reading drafts of this book and to encourage me along the way.

Eleanor Carey, Barbara Dunne and Emer Henry are close friends of Emer's and mine and were a very important source of friendship and support to Emer in her tough days. We have known each other since we were 18 and have always been in each other's lives.

Noeleen Kavanagh, Anne Marie Sullivan and Emer O'Neill were school friends of Emer's. They stayed close to Emer through thick and thin and have each stayed in touch with me and Clodagh and Ronan since Emer died.

Emer was especially close to Mary Ward and Annette Rhatigan, two wonderful women who were also public health doctors. They made work fun and bearable for Emer. And I know there were others who also did so, like Fiona Cloak. I'm grateful to them all for all they did for Emer and for staying in touch.

Ronan has two friends, both called Max – Russell and Fitzgerald – he has known since Montessori. They come from great families, and both their mums, Ailish and Carole, were fantastic. You could pick up the phone at any time and ask them for anything. They would drop in and out to Emer, go to the pharmacy for her, give lifts, pick up kids, etc. That kind of practical support was invaluable, and I recall it so gratefully. It is what allows you to function and keep all the balls in the air.

Emer was cared for expertly and compassionately by Professor Paul Browne and Dr Norma O'Leary, both of whom will forever have a special place in our hearts. Paul is a man of great emotional intelligence in whom Emer had complete faith. He gave us the gift of life. He enabled Emer to see Clodagh and Ronan into adulthood. Emer could not have survived for so long without his expert care. Norma O'Leary provided expert comfort and care to Emer over the eight years of her illness. Her humanity made the unbearable bearable for Emer and for our family. There were many other doctors, nurses and other staff who cared for Emer in St James's Hospital and Our Lady's Hospice in Harold's Cross. Dr Barry Quinn, who is a good friend, was also a wonderful GP for Emer from the start of her illness. He is everything you would want in a GP – expert, compassionate and committed.

Tina Pluck was also a great support and friend to Emer and to our family and I am happy that she is still in our lives more than 20 years after Martha introduced us.

Emer's morning and evening home care visits in the period before she died were provided by two wonderful women called Suzanne and Martina. Suzanne and Emer had a similarly wicked sense of humour, and they formed a close bond in a very short space of time. Suzanne was there every morning and evening to help Emer. We had converted a TV room downstairs into a bedroom, and when I think back to that time, what I remember is the sound of Emer and Suzanne laughing and joking together.

While Emer was isolated in St James's Hospital for her transplant in 2013 one other point of contact was a wonderful woman called Joan, who would come in and out, clean the room, bring Emer food, and chat to her about her own life, which was 'real life'. Everything else was clinical and sanitised and medical. Joan was a lifeline, and Emer never forgot her kindness. Sister Joyce Cullinane was an ever-present pastor, friend and source of joy who always lifted Emer's spirits. Father John Browne touched Emer's soul in a special way and led the celebration of her life with warmth, insight and consideration.

The project to transform the garden while Emer was having her stem cell transplant was carried out by my good friend, Charlie Roarty, a proud Donegal man from Gweedore with a big heart and a soft voice. One of the best men you could come across. He was a contractor on small domestic projects, mostly in our neighbourhood. We got to know each other through GAA commitments. He arrived to do the job as soon as Emer left for the hospital and he hardly left until he finished it – on time, on budget and to the highest of standards with a team of lovely men with Donegal accents. Alongside the garden project, Peter Hintz, a Polish man with a great sense of humour and wit, put everything aside to prioritise painting the house from top to bottom while Emer was in hospital. I want Charlie and Peter to know these were much more than projects to us. Emer derived happiness and comfort from their work for many years.

Ballybunion was a special place for the Feely family for over forty years. It became a central part of my life with Emer and of our children's lives. It is a wonderful place of natural beauty and, much more important, a place of warm-hearted, witty and welcoming people. We were overwhelmed to see the picture of the sand art tribute to Emer on the Ladies' Beach on the day that she died. It meant so much to our family.

To all our friends, neighbours and especially Denis Boland, chairman, and everyone in Templeogue Synge Street GAA club, thank you for your patience, understanding and kindness over many tough years and for always lending an empathetic ear.

In my years in the Department of Health, I met some of the best people I've ever worked with. Tracey Conroy and Fergal Goodman were two of the best. Passionate, committed and idealistic, full of integrity and ambitious for health and improved services, I am happy to say they are lifelong friends. I learned so much from them over many years of working closely together. We each progressed to join the management board. We each benefited from knowing each other and working closely together. Tracey was a source of good counsel, strength and loyal friendship through difficult times. I won't forget that.

Thankfully I had Pauline Brady, my loyal PA and friend, through all my time as CMO. If it weren't for her, I wouldn't have been able to do half the job I did. I don't think she knows how much I valued her constant support and help, personally and professionally. She was later joined by Helen Reddin. Initially Pauline and I were both concerned about how it would work if she had to share an office – she had been alone for so long. But we need not have feared. Helen brought the same standard of commitment and loyalty. She and Pauline became great friends and remain so even though promotion for each of them has taken them to different sections in the department.

Pauline and Helen were very supportive during the pandemic, including many long and heavy NPHET meetings which I chaired from my office over a computer screen. They would appear in my room with coffee or a small snack to keep me going. There were definitely days when all I wanted to do at the end of a NPHET meeting was lie down in a dark room! But I never did. The usual arrangement was to grab a quick bite and then meet the minister to take him through the new advice that would be in the NPHET letter. In this regard, thanks is due to the unseen work of the secretariat team that expertly supported the NPHET. The pressure was on them to turn around detailed letters of advice for issue to the minister, and to a high standard, within hours of the end of each meeting. It was a tough but important task and I really valued and trusted the team who had that responsibility.

The NPHET process served the country well, in my opinion. I will always be grateful to the members for their selfless contribution over such a long period of time and their willingness to always respond to a call to attend, no matter the impact on their personal lives. The members were chosen as leaders in their own fields of expertise of responsibility and they made that available for the common good. With their commitment and forbearance, we overcame the limitations of having to work for most of the time through a virtual process. I thank the members for their patience and understanding of the impact it placed on how we operated as a team.

We had a wonderful press and communications team during the pandemic, headed by Deirdre Watters and including especially Aoife Gilligan, Lindsay Drea, Sinéad O'Donnell, Fiona Hyde, Ailish Murray and Róisín Collier. There were others too. The entire team were expert, professional, enthusiastic and wholly committed to what we were doing. They were always aware of what was under discussion in the media and on social media, and would tell me at a moment's notice what I needed to know. I trusted that. Fully.

Many of the members of the NPHET also participated in the daily EpiCall meeting. These included the deputy CMOs in my division, including Dr Ronan Glynn, Dr Alan Smith, Dr Eibhlín Connolly, Dr Colette Bonner and Dr Darina O'Flanagan. The EpiCall also included the press and communications team, Philip Nolan as chair of the 'modelling' team and the statistics team of Ronan O'Kelly, Shona Gilsenan and Pauline White in the Department of Health. It also included great colleagues like Laura Casey, who worked on developing the detailed policy and strategy to respond on behalf of and to be approved by the NPHET and Dr Siobhán O'Sullivan, the Chief Bioethics Officer. Key members of Fergal Goodman's and Tracey Conroy's divisions were also included.

Ronan Glynn is someone to whom I owe an enormous debt of gratitude. He stepped in to take on responsibility for leading the pandemic response when Emer was admitted to hospice care in July 2020 and again when she died in February 2021. I first met Ronan some years earlier when he came to my office on the public health training programme. In fact, he had worked with Emer in the HSE prior to joining my office and I remember her saying to me, 'You're getting a really good guy next.' How right she was. In time, he was appointed as a deputy CMO. From the outset, he had my trust and confidence and I never came to doubt that early judgement. He will have a special place in our family story because it was his willingness and ability in stepping into my role that enabled me to step back when Emer needed it.

I thank all of the people I worked with over many years in the Department of Health and the wider health system. I was lucky to have had many great people in my team and in the division I led. I am proud of the many things we managed to achieve together. I am proud of having worked with them all. Siobhán O'Sullivan, Claire Gordon, Kathleen MacLellan and Kate O'Flaherty are shining stars in that regard.

As I move on to life beyond the Department of Health, I have many people to thank. Dermot McCrum has been a trusted adviser and manager. We have known each other for twenty years and he has helped and advised me on various projects, which has been invaluable to me. Professor Cecily Kelleher and the College of Health and Agricultural Sciences in UCD appointed me as Adjunct Full Professor of Public Health. Linda Doyle, Provost of Trinity College Dublin, believed in my vision for a role which unfortunately, through no fault of hers, has not happened. I thank Louis Ronan for the opportunity to advise his new company, Enfer Medical. I thank Jean Callinan, chair, and all my fellow board members for the privilege of joining the board of the Irish Hospice Foundation and being able to support the work of its staff.

I have also found time in this new life to work on some new and exciting projects, which will hopefully bear fruit in the future, with some wonderful new friends including Shane Gillen, Una Molloy and Greg O'Donoghue.

I thank Hans Kluge, Gabrielle Jacob, Hande Harmanci, Ibrahim Durak and others in the WHO European headquarters in Copenhagen and the Country Office in Baku, Azerbaijan for the opportunity to work with them as an external consultant.

When it comes to this book, writing it has been an enormously enjoyable experience. But I know myself well enough to know that I would not have managed it without the patient expertise, professionalism and humanity of Emily Hourican, who wrote it with me. She never once showed any impatience as I hacked at her work and as I changed my mind as we went from draft to draft. It was simply a pleasure to work with her.

Marianne Gunne O'Connor is my agent. I am so fortunate to have such a credible, expert and experienced guide as I take on a project such as this. She arranged meetings with a number of publishers and advised on the selection of Bonnier/Eriu to publish the book.

That proved a great decision. I am honoured to work with Deirdre Nolan, whose late father was a teacher in my secondary school. Her editorial expertise and dedication have transformed my words into this story.

I am deeply indebted to those people close to me who read drafts of the book as it evolved and added value to the product it now is. They were Ciara Cronin, Orla Feely, Aileen Holohan, Colin Doherty and Dermot McCrum.